71

THE
WATERCRESS
SOUP DIET

'It's fatless, low calorie, full of vitamins and iron and delicious enough to serve at a dinner party. I drink at least six cups a day when eager to lose pounds.'
LIZ HURLEY

THE
WATERCRESS
SOUP DIET

MARIANNE DAWSON

JB

JOHN BLAKE

Published by John Blake Publishing Ltd,
3 Bramber Court, 2 Bramber Road,
London W14 9PB, England

First published in paperback 2002

ISBN 1903402 73 5

British Library Cataloguing-in-Publication Data:

A catalogue record for this book is
available from the British Library.

Design by NV

Printed in Great Britain by
Bookmarque

1 3 5 7 9 10 8 6 4 2

Papers used by John Blake Publishing Limited are natural,
recyclable products made from wood grown in sustainable forests.
The manufacturing processes conform to the environmental
regulations of the country of origin.

IMPORTANT NOTE

The Watercress Soup Diet is an incredibly intensive weight-loss plan. Over the period of just a week, you can easily lose up to ten pounds.

However, it is not designed to be used for more than a week, and is not intended as a substitute for a long-term eating plan. In Part 3 of this book, you will find a number of balanced, low-calorie daily menus. These are intended to help you develop a sensible, lasting approach to eating. You may only return to the Watercress Soup Diet after a break of four weeks.

The reader should consult his or her doctor before embarking upon this diet, especially if he or she is currently undergoing any kind of medication.

The Watercress Soup Diet is under no circumstances suitable for children.

contents

part ❶

part ❷

RECIPE SUGGESTIONS FOR THE WATERCRESS SOUP DIET

part ❸

KEEPING WEIGHT OFF –
THE FOLLOW-ON DIET

part ❹

ENTERTAINING ON THE DIET

part ❺

DIETING TIPS 172

introduction

WHAT IS THE WATERCRESS SOUP DIET?

Congratulations! On buying this book, you have taken the first step in revolutionising your life and achieving the weight you've been aiming for. The Watercress Soup Diet is a quick, safe and easy way of losing weight, and most importantly, keeping it off.

The Watercress Soup Diet itself is a one-week diet plan that aims to help you lose ten pounds over seven days. The beauty of the diet is that it doesn't involve you having to starve yourself. Everything is very carefully balanced so that you can eat as much as you like of tasty, healthy foods. The biggest barrier most people find to losing weight is the discomfort of hunger pangs. With the Watercress Soup Diet, they simply won't arise.

WHY WATERCRESS?

The beauty of the Watercress Soup Diet is that not only is the soup that forms its basis incredibly tasty, it's also really good for you. Watercress is a genuine superfood! It's packed full of vitamins A, B and C, plus iron, folic acid and many minerals. Perhaps more importantly, it is a rich source of 'antioxidants'. These mop up harmful free radicals, atoms that damage DNA and cause cells to become cancerous. Indeed, it is as an anti-cancer dietary source that watercress is of such interest to food researchers.

The values of watercress have been understood for many years. Over the centuries it has been an official medicine, even during the days of the ancient Greeks. Hippocrates, who is often thought of as the father of medicine, is understood to have chosen the location of his first hospital on the basis of its proximity to a stream that was a good source of the plant. For hundreds of years, watercress has been used as a cure for anaemia, in poultices for inflammation, and even as an antiseptic.

In 19th-century England, watercress was the staple of the working classes, and was most often eaten for breakfast in a sandwich. If the family was too poor to buy bread, they would often substitute raw watercress instead, and so the plant became known as 'poor man's bread'. Soon it was grown commercially in the chalk streams of Hampshire and Dorset, from where it was taken up to Covent Garden to be sold. Street-vendors would sell it in bunches to be eaten hand-held – it was even reputed then, as it is now, to be a good cure for a hangover! (Unfortunately, you won't be able to try this out during the week-long Watercress Soup Diet, as alcohol, I'm afraid, is out!)

So you see, eating watercress can only do you good! As well as the watercress in the soup, I have tried to include as much of this amazing plant as possible in the other recipes that you will find in this book.

HOW IS THIS BOOK DIVIDED UP?

There are five parts to this book. They are as follows:

Part One – The Watercress Soup Diet
This is where it all starts! You will find a detailed, day-by-day list of what you are allowed to eat on

the diet. You may be surprised to see that you can eat all sorts of foods – including chicken and fish – and of course as much as you like of the delicious watercress soup! Follow this part carefully, and you'll literally see the pounds drop off....

Part Two – Recipe Suggestions for the Watercress Soup Diet

Because the food you can eat on the diet is so varied, there are loads of different recipes you can prepare whilst you're shedding the pounds. In Part 2, you will find a list of ideas for how to make your diet quite delicious!

Part Three – Keeping Weight Off – The Follow-On Diet

OK, so you've lost more weight than you'd thought possible in a week. The big question is – how do you keep it off? You can't keep doing the Watercress Soup Diet for ever – it's such an intensive weight-loss programme that it cannot safely be done for more than a week at a time (although you can go back to it after a four-week break). Part 3 outlines a brand new, low-calorie weight-loss plan that is very low in fat – but I think you'll be surprised by how versatile and delicious it is.

Part Four – Entertaining on the Diet
Just because you're dieting, it doesn't mean you can't enjoy yourself. This section gives you six sensational dinner party menus that you can serve your guests – and they'll never even know you're on a diet!

Part Five – Dieting Tips
Successful weight loss is not just a matter of what you eat. In Part 5 you'll find 50 essential tips to help you slim down and look good.

So, now you know what you are about to embark upon, let's get stuck in, shall we?

KEY
For those of you who are not natural cooks, here's a quick guide to a few of the culinary terms that you'll encounter in this book:

dsp	level dessertspoon(ful)
fl oz	fluid ounces
l	litres
ml	millilitre
tbsp	level tablespoon(ful)
tsp	level teaspoon(ful)

part 1

the watercress soup diet

THE MOST IMPORTANT BIT – HOW DO I MAKE WATERCRESS SOUP?

If you look through your recipe books, you'll find any number of recipes for watercress soup. Some of them are straightforward, some of them are quite complicated; some are high in calories, others less so. That is why it is recommended that you use this version if you are to lose weight at the rate that you want. It's really easy to make, and it's very low in calories, which means that you can drink as much of it as you like, whenever you get a hunger pang during the week of the diet. So here goes:

WATERCRESS SOUP

1 small onion, finely chopped
2½ pints of light chicken stock or water
2 small potatoes, diced
3 large bunches of watercress, stems removed
salt and pepper

Sweat the onion in two or three tablespoons of chicken stock or water. Add the potatoes together with the seasoning and the stock. Bring to the boil and simmer until the potatoes are soft. Add the watercress, and stir for three minutes. Remove from the heat and blend in a liquidiser.

At this point, put the soup in a metal bowl and place it in a sink full of ice-cold water. This will keep the lovely green colour of the soup and make it even more appetising. The soup is delicious drunk cold, but you can also heat it up if you wish to have it nice and hot.

HOW THE DIET WORKS

The Watercress Soup Diet is not difficult, but it must

be strictly adhered to. I'll reiterate that it is a very intensive weight-loss programme, but it *does* have to be followed accurately to produce results.

The first thing to say is that you are allowed to eat as much of the watercress soup as you want, at any time of the day, on any day of the week. Don't go mad, but whenever you feel yourself getting hungry between meals, have a quick bowl of the soup and your hunger pangs will soon disappear.

But there is much more to the diet than just watercress soup. Indeed, on most days, you are allowed to eat as much as you want of certain foods – and not just boring foods either! Chicken is on the menu, as is fish, and loads of fruit and vegetables. A lot of people who follow the diet actually find that it gets them to change their eating habits almost immediately – the food really does taste that good.

Let's start by looking at exactly what you are allowed to eat on each of the seven days of the diet.

DAY 1

1. Unlimited watercress soup
2. Fruit from the Watercress Soup Diet Fruit List
3. 250ml skimmed milk or fat-free yoghurt

DAY 2

1. Unlimited watercress soup
2. Vegetables from the Watercress Soup Diet Vegetable List
3. 1 jacket potato
4. 250ml skimmed milk or fat-free yoghurt

DAY 3

1. Unlimited watercress soup
2. Fruit from the Watercress Soup Diet Fruit List
3. Vegetables from the Watercress Soup Diet Vegetable List
4. 250ml skimmed milk or fat-free yoghurt

DAY 4

1. Unlimited watercress soup
2. 5 bananas
3. 8 x 250ml servings of skimmed milk (you may, if you wish, replace one – but only one – of these servings of milk with a 250ml serving of fat-free yoghurt)

DAY 5

1. Unlimited watercress soup
2. As much white fish as you need to satisfy your hunger without overeating

3. As much skinless, lean chicken as you need to satisfy your hunger without overeating
4. Up to 6 fresh tomatoes, or 1 tin of tomatoes
5. 250ml skimmed milk or fat-free yoghurt

DAY 6

1. Unlimited watercress soup
2. As much white fish as you need to satisfy your hunger without overeating
3. As much skinless, lean chicken as you need to satisfy your hunger without overeating
4. Vegetables from the Watercress Soup Diet Vegetable List, including tomatoes
5. 250ml skimmed milk or fat-free yoghurt

DAY 7

1. Unlimited watercress soup
2. Fruit from the Watercress Soup Diet Fruit List
3. Vegetables from the Watercress Soup Diet Vegetable List
4. 250ml skimmed milk or fat-free yoghurt

You see what I mean when I said it was simple?

A FEW SIMPLE RULES

As you can see, on certain days you can eat as much of certain foods as you want – fruit and vegetables from the Watercress Soup Diet lists to be found on page 26, for example; even, on days five and six, an unlimited quantity of fish and chicken. Now, although it is true that you can eat as much as you like of these foods, and still succeed in your weight-loss programme, it is very important that you try not to overeat. Always remember that if you are going to keep the weight off that you have lost as a result of this diet, you are going to have to curb any desires you might have to overeat. Your new way of eating starts here!

You must also remember that, just as it is important not to overdo things, it is equally important not to skip foods. Every food on the Watercress Soup Diet is there for a reason. Each contains a necessary quantity of certain nutrients and minerals that you need in order to eat healthily. The banana frenzy on Day 4, for example, is designed to ensure that your potassium levels are kept up, and the milk is there to make sure that you don't lose out on your all-important calcium intake.

FLAVOURINGS

You are allowed to use flavourings or condiments, but only if they contain less than 25 calories per teaspoon. Here are a few suggestions:

- Japanese rice vinegar
- Lemon juice with a little sweetener and chopped mint
- Orange juice and chopped mint
- 2 tbsps white wine vinegar, 1 tsp Dijon mustard and 1 tsp hot horseradish
- Japanese all-purpose soya

MILK OR YOGHURT?

It is very important to remember that you cannot combine milk and yoghurt during the same day. You must decide at the beginning of each day whether you are going to drink milk or eat yoghurt...

You can, of course, drink as much water as you like during the week – in fact, it is positively recommended. Try and drink a pint of water first thing in the morning, and drink as much as you can throughout the day. Did you know that top supermodels drink iced water all the time because it makes their bodies burn up calories to warm it up? As far as other drinks are concerned, you may drink as much black tea or coffee as you want (sweetened only with artificial, low-calorie sweetener); but it is a good health tip, whether you are dieting or not, to drink two glasses of water for every cup of tea or coffee that you consume. Don't worry about the water making you feel bloated – it is only when you don't drink enough water that you suffer from water retention. Try and drink at least a couple of litres a day.

THE FRUIT AND VEGETABLE LISTS

Looking at the diet plan, you will see that on different days you are allowed to eat as much as you like of certain fruits and vegetables. Note that you cannot eat any old fruit or vegetable, as some are more conducive to the kind of high-speed weight loss we are trying to achieve than others. Don't worry though – there are plenty to chose from!

Note that although tomatoes are available on days 5 and 6, they are not listed here, as you can't eat them every day.

THE WATERCRESS SOUP DIET VEGETABLE LIST

Artichokes	Courgettes
Asparagus	Cucumber
Aubergine	Lettuce
Beans	Mushrooms
Beetroot	Onions
Broccoli	Parsley
Brussels Sprouts	Peppers
Cabbage	Radishes
Carrots	Spinach
Cauliflower	Turnip
Celery	Watercress (of course!)

THE WATERCRESS SOUP DIET FRUIT LIST

Apples	Melons
Apricots	Nectarines
Berries	Oranges
Blueberries	Peaches
Cherries	Pineapple
Grapefruit	Plums
Grapes	Raspberries
Kiwi Fruit	Strawberries
Lemons	Tangerines

THE INGREDIENTS TABLE

This table details exactly what you can eat on which day. You will find copies of it starting on page 185. All you need to do is cross off what you have eaten on any particular day, to make sure that you are a) eating the right things, and b) not eating too much of certain foods. In the milk and yoghurt row, cross off each unit of 25ml of milk/yoghurt that you have consumed, apart from on Day 4, when you can cross off each unit of 250ml you have consumed. Remember, you can only have milk or yoghurt on each particular day, apart from Day 4 when you can replace one of your portions of milk with a portion of yoghurt.

part 2

recipe suggestions for the watercress soup diet

OK, so now you understand the diet. You could just go ahead and pick and mix allowable foods on each day, and you'll watch the pounds drop off. But the beauty of the Watercress Soup Diet is its versatility. There are so many good things you can eat during the course of the week-long programme, this is one of the few diets that really don't have to be boring.

In this section, I have suggested a few simple recipes for each day of the diet. You can eat as much as you like of most of these recipes, but do remember to keep an eye on your milk or yoghurt intake: it is important that you do not exceed this. I have indicated in the recipe if you are using a proportion of your milk or yoghurt allowance, and if so, how much. Enjoy!

POSSIBLE RECIPES FOR DAY 1

SUMMER YOGHURT

Serves 1

> 60g strawberries
> 60g raspberries
> 250ml low-fat natural yoghurt

Purée the strawberries and raspberries, mix with the yoghurt and serve.

You could also eat this on days 3 and 7

CINNAMON GRAPEFRUIT

Serves 1

> ½ grapefruit
> ¼ tsp cinnamon
> ¼ tsp ground ginger
> a sprig of ginger mint

Place the grapefruit under a medium grill until it begins to bubble and go brown. Sprinkle with the spices, and serve garnished with the mint.

You could also eat this on days 3 and 7

RECIPE SUGGESTIONS FOR THE WATERCRESS SOUP DIET

BLUEBERRY BAKED APPLE

Serves 1

1 large apple
1 dsp blueberries
1 tsp sweetener
½ tsp cinnamon

Pre-heat the oven to 175°C. Core the apple. Put in an ovenproof dish with a little water. Mix the berries, sweetener and cinnamon together, and put the mixture inside the apple. Bake until soft. You could also cook this in the microwave – check the manufacturer's instructions for the exact timing.

You could also eat this on days 3 and 7

STRAWBERRY MILKSHAKE WITH A DIFFERENCE

What's the difference? A twist of pepper, which sounds strange but really brings out the taste of the strawberries...

Serves 1

    1 small punnet strawberries
    a couple of turns of black pepper
    250ml skimmed milk

Blitz all the ingredients in a liquidiser and serve.

NB: This recipe uses your entire daily milk allowance.

You could also eat this on days 3 and 7

MINTY GRILLED PINEAPPLE

Serves 1

    60ml orange juice
    1/2 a fresh pineapple
    2 tsp fresh mint, chopped

Skin, slice and core the pineapple, then grill it under a medium grill until nicely caramelised. Heat the orange juice, and serve the pineapple with the juice poured over it and sprinkled with fresh mint.

You could also eat this on days 3 and 7

RECIPE SUGGESTIONS FOR THE WATERCRESS SOUP DIET

FRUIT SALAD

Serves 1–2

1 slice honeydew melon, cut into chunks
1 nectarine, stoned and sliced
½ tangerine, segmented
½ apple, cored and chopped
8 strawberries, sliced
6 seedless green grapes
juice of 1 orange
1 dsp fresh mint, chopped

Combine the melon, nectarine, tangerine, apple, strawberries and grapes in a serving bowl. Mix the orange juice and mint, and pour over the fruit before serving.

You could also eat this on days 3 and 7

POSSIBLE RECIPES FOR DAY 2

CHILLED CUCUMBER AND LEMON SOUP

Serves 1

> 1 medium-sized cucumber
> 120ml low-fat natural yoghurt
> 1 small clove garlic, crushed
> salt and freshly ground black pepper
> 1 tsp lemon juice
> 1 tsp fresh garden mint, chopped
> a few slices of lemon, cut very thinly

Peel the cucumber thinly, leaving a little of the green, then slice it. Keep a few thinly cut slices as a garnish. Liquidise the rest of the cucumber with the yoghurt and crushed garlic. Blend until the mixture is smooth. Add the salt, pepper and lemon juice. If the soup appears to be too thick at this stage, you can thin it with some vegetable stock. Stir in the chopped mint, cover and chill for a few hours. Serve with the slices of cucumber and lemon on each portion.

NB: This recipe uses nearly half of your daily yoghurt allowance.

You can also eat this on days 3, 6 and 7

RECIPE SUGGESTIONS FOR THE WATERCRESS SOUP DIET

CRUNCHY SPINACH SALAD

Serves 1

  3 handfuls baby spinach, stalks removed
  1 punnet small cress
  $1/4$ cucumber
  2 tsp lemon juice
  $1/2$ tsp French mustard
  a little vegetable stock, if needed
  6 radishes, sliced

Wash the spinach and cress, dry carefully and mix together on a large plate. Peel the cucumber and then liquidise with the lemon juice and mustard. If too thick, add a little vegetable stock. Pour over the salad, and garnish with the radishes.

You can also eat this on days 3, 6 and 7

BAKED POTATO WITH ROASTED VEGETABLES

Serves 1

  1 large baked potato
  the white part of a small leek, sliced thinly
  1 spring onion, sliced
  $1/4$ pepper, sliced
  1 tbsp low-fat dressing (I recommend Japanese
  seasoned rice vinegar – available at Sainsbury's)
  salt and freshly ground black pepper

Bake the leek, onion and pepper until slightly charred. Mix with the dressing, season to taste, and spoon over the potato.

WARM RUBY SALAD WITH ROSEMARY

Serves 4

6 medium red onions, peeled and quartered
4 large sprigs rosemary
3 medium beetroot, peeled and quartered
450ml vegetable stock
2 tbsp raspberry vinegar
salt and freshly ground black pepper
1 tbsp low-fat natural yoghurt
rosemary sprigs to garnish

Partially cook the onions in the microwave with the rosemary, covered. Put the stock and vinegar in a pan, add the beetroot and onions with the rosemary. Bring to the boil and simmer for one hour until the beetroot is tender. Remove the lid and boil steadily until the liquid reduces to a glaze. Season and discard the rosemary. Transfer to a warm serving dish, spoon the yoghurt over, and garnish with rosemary sprigs.

NB: This recipe uses 1 tbsp of your daily yoghurt allowance.

You can also eat this on days 3, 6 and 7

BAKED POTATO WITH WATERCRESS AND SPINACH

Serves 1

1 large baked potato
1 tbsp low-fat yoghurt
1 tsp celery leaves, chopped
1 tsp chives, chopped
2 small handfuls watercress
1 small handful spinach
a little lemon juice
salt and freshly ground black pepper

Combine the yoghurt, celery leaves and chives. Season well. Make a salad of the watercress and spinach, and use a little lemon juice as a dressing. Spoon the yoghurt mixture over the potato, and serve with the salad on one side.

NB: This recipe uses 1 tbsp of your daily yoghurt allowance.

CHINESE MIXED VEGETABLES

Serves 2

> 1 large carrot, peeled and cut into batons
> 1 courgette, peeled and cut into batons
> 2 sticks celery, trimmed and cut into batons
> 1 leek, cut into ½-inch pieces
> a small piece of ginger, peeled and sliced
> 2 tbsp soy sauce
> 1 tsp five-spice powder
> juice and grated rind of ½ lime
> salt and freshly ground pepper
> 1 dsp fresh coriander, chopped

Cook the vegetables in the microwave until they are cooked through, but retain some bite. In the meantime, mix the ginger and spices into the soy sauce. Add the rind and juice of the lime. Pour over the hot vegetables and toss. Garnish with chopped coriander.

You can also eat this on days 3, 6 and 7

RECIPE SUGGESTIONS FOR THE WATERCRESS SOUP DIET

POSSIBLE RECIPES FOR DAY 3

HOT CITRUS SALAD

Serves 1

  1 orange, peeled and segmented
  1 pink grapefruit, peeled and segmented
  1 tangerine, peeled and segmented

Pre-heat the oven to 175°C. Place all the ingredients in an ovenproof dish. Bake in the oven for about ten minutes, and serve piping hot.

You can also eat this on Day 7

GRILLED APRICOTS WITH ORANGE DRESSING

Serves 1

  2–3 apricots
  90ml fresh orange juice

Halve the apricots and remove the stones. Place under a medium grill until nicely caramelised. In the meantime, heat the orange juice. Serve the apricots with the juice poured over, and sprinkled with a little sweetener if desired.

You can also eat this on Day 7

BRAISED CELERY HEARTS

Serves 2

1 heart of celery, trimmed, cleaned and cut in
  half
segments cut from 1 large orange, rind and pith
  removed
juice of ½ orange
60ml vegetable stock
1 tsp fresh rosemary, chopped

Place the prepared celery in a suitable microwave
dish, together with the orange segments, orange
juice and stock. Cook until tender. Sprinkle with the
rosemary before serving.

You can also eat this on Day 7

SALAD OF ASPARAGUS AND LAMB'S LETTUCE

Serves 1

6 stalks asparagus
1 courgette
2 tbsp vegetable stock
1 tbsp lemon juice
salt and freshly ground black pepper
lamb's lettuce

Gently scrape the stems of the asparagus. Place them in a pan of cold water, bring to the boil, and cook until tender.

To make a courgette purée, peel and slice the courgette, and cook gently in the stock. Liquidise, adding lemon juice, salt and pepper to taste. Leave to cool. Place the courgette purée in the middle of a plate, top with the cold asparagus, and surround with lamb's lettuce.

You can also eat this on days 2, 6 and 7

ARTICHOKE HEARTS AUX FINES HERBES

Serves 1

4 tinned artichoke hearts
juice of ½ lemon
a little stock
1 tbsp fresh mixed herbs, chopped

Place three of the artichoke hearts on a plate and sprinkle with a little lemon juice. Liquidise the remaining heart with the rest of the lemon juice and enough stock to make a pouring consistency. Add the chopped herbs, pour over the artichoke hearts.

You can also eat this on days 2, 6 and 7

SURPRISE SALAD

Serves 2

1/2 oak leaf lettuce
2 ripe peaches, halved, stoned and thinly sliced
a 2-inch piece of cucumber, thinly sliced
1/2 red pepper, halved, de-seeded and thinly
   sliced
90g mushroom caps, cleaned and thinly sliced
90g carrot, peeled and finely grated
12 seedless black grapes
1 dsp fresh herbs, chopped

For the Peach Dressing

1 ripe peach
1 tsp prepared English mustard
1 1/2 tbsp white wine vinegar

First make the dressing. Gently poach the peach in a
little water until soft. Liquidise with the mustard and
vinegar. Heat, and keep warm. Meanwhile, place the
salad ingredients in layers in a salad bowl, with the
lettuce leaves on the bottom. Pour the warm
dressing over, and garnish with the fresh herbs.

You can also eat this on Day 7

POSSIBLE RECIPES FOR DAY 4

BANANA SMOOTHIE

Serves 1

1 banana
250ml skimmed milk

Blitz the banana and the milk together in a liquidiser. Pour into a cold glass and serve.

NB: This recipe uses one of your 8 x 250ml milk allowances.

BANANA MOUSSE

Serves 1

1/2 vanilla pod
2 bananas
125ml yoghurt

Remove the seeds from the vanilla pod. Mash the seeds well with the bananas, and fold into the yoghurt. Could there be an easier recipe?

NB: This recipe uses half your daily yoghurt allowance.

JACKET BANANA

Serves 1

1 banana

Pre-heat the oven to 175°C. Bake the banana for 15 minutes or until soft. The skin will go black. When cooked, remove from the oven, make an incision along the length of the banana and eat from the skin with a teaspoon.

EXOTIC YOGHURT DRINK

Serves 1

250ml low-fat natural yoghurt
250ml skimmed milk
4 drops rose-water
1/2 tsp ground cardamom
1/2 tsp cinnamon
a little sweetener
60ml cold water
4 ice cubes

Place all the ingredients in a liquidiser. Liquidise, and pour into a tall glass. Serve chilled.

NB: Day 4 is the only day when you can have milk and yoghurt. This recipe uses your daily yoghurt allowance, and one of your remaining seven daily milk allowances.

POSSIBLE RECIPES FOR DAY 5

VANILLA MILK WARMER

Serves 1

    250ml skimmed milk
    a few drops vanilla extract
    1/4 tsp ground nutmeg

Heat the milk and vanilla together. Transfer to a cup and sprinkle the nutmeg on top. Serve hot.

This recipe can be used on any day

SPICY TOMATO JUICE

Serves 2

    6 tomatoes, chopped
    60 ml water
    small stick of celery
    1/2 bay leaf
    2 sprigs parsley
    2 sprigs basil
    a pinch of salt
    a pinch of paprika
    a dash of Worcestershire sauce
    a couple of drops of Tabasco sauce
    a squeeze of lemon juice

Place the tomatoes, water, celery, bay leaf, parsley and basil in a saucepan and simmer until the tomatoes are nice and soft. Strain through a sieve, and season with the salt, paprika, Worcestershire sauce, Tabasco and lemon juice. Serve cold.

This recipe can also be used on Day 6

FISH KEBABS ON A BED OF WATERCRESS

Serves 1

  240g halibut
  6 cherry tomatoes
  4 bay leaves
  2 kebab skewers
  a good handful of watercress
  lemon juice

Cut the halibut into bite-sized pieces. Thread the fish, tomatoes and bay leaves onto the skewers, alternating each ingredient along the skewer. Grill until the tomatoes are soft and the fish cooked through. Dress the watercress with the lemon juice, arrange on a plate, lay the kebabs on top and serve.

This recipe can also be used on Day 6

ROSEMARY-INFUSED CHICKEN KEBABS

Serves 1

- 240g chicken breast, skin removed
- 8 cherry tomatoes
- a few bay leaves, fresh if you have them
- 2 strong rosemary stalks, leaves removed (or kebab skewers)
- 2 ripe tomatoes
- a few basil leaves
- 1 tbsp low-calorie dressing

For the Marinade

- 1 tbsp low-fat natural yoghurt
- 1 tsp lemon juice
- salt and freshly ground black pepper
- ½ tsp dried mixed herbs

Chop the chicken breast into bite-sized pieces. Mix the marinade ingredients together and then add the pieces of chicken. Put in the fridge for 2 hours. Thread the chicken, cherry tomatoes and bay leaves onto the rosemary stalks or kebab skewers, and grill until the chicken is cooked. In the meantime, slice the remaining tomatoes and make a salad with the dressing and the basil leaves. Serve the kebabs with the tomato salad.

This recipe can also be used on Day 6

CHICKEN IN A PARCEL

Serves 1

  1 x 240g breast of chicken, skin removed
  4 tomatoes, sliced
  1 dsp lemon juice
  1 tsp fresh thyme, chopped
  a few chives, chopped
  a few basil leaves
  1 tbsp low-calorie dressing
  salt and freshly ground black pepper

Pre-heat the oven to 190°C. Cut a square of parchment baking paper (available from any good supermarket) large enough to wrap around the chicken piece loosely. Take two of the sliced tomatoes and place them in the centre of the paper. Season with salt and pepper. Place the chicken on top of the tomatoes, and sprinkle with lemon juice, thyme and chives. Wrap the parchment around the chicken, and scrunch up at the top so that no steam will escape. Place on a baking tray and bake for about 20 minutes, or until the chicken is cooked. Serve with a salad made of the remaining tomatoes, basil leaves, dressing, salt and pepper.

This recipe can also be used on Day 6

COD GRILLED WITH TOMATOES AND LEMON

Serves 1

2 tomatoes
1 x 8oz fillet of cod
juice of 1 lemon

Pre-heat the oven to 190°C. Put the tomatoes in an ovenproof dish and cook for about 15 minutes or until cooked. Smear the fish with the lemon juice. Grill carefully on both sides until just cooked. Serve with the baked tomatoes, and any juices from the fish.

This recipe can also be used on Day 6

POSSIBLE RECIPES FOR DAY 6

CHILLED SALAD OF MEDITERRANEAN VEGETABLES

Serves 2

240g ripe tomatoes, skinned
½ large green pepper
½ large yellow pepper
¼ small cucumber
2 small cloves garlic
3 tbsp tomato juice
1 tbsp red wine vinegar
a good pinch cayenne pepper or chilli powder
a few radishes, cut into quarters
salt and freshly ground black pepper

Core and dice the peeled tomatoes into ½-inch cubes. De-seed the peppers and cut them into thin strips. Cut the cucumber into strips of the same size. Make the dressing by combining the garlic, tomato juice, vinegar, cayenne pepper or chilli powder, salt and pepper. Arrange the vegetables on a serving dish, pour over a small amount of the dressing, then chill for 30 minutes. Remove the chilled salad from the fridge and pour the remaining dressing over it. Garnish with the radishes.

STUFFED TOMATOES

2 shallots
60g button mushrooms
1 tbsp lemon juice
1 tsp fresh herbs, chopped
2 tsp tomato ketchup
2 large tomatoes
a few chopped chives

Pre-heat the oven to 175°C. Chop the shallots and mushrooms finely, and cook gently in a little lemon juice. Add the chopped herbs and the ketchup. Cut the tops off the tomatoes and spoon out the seeds and juice. Fill the cavities with the mixture and bake for 15–20 minutes. Serve garnished with chopped chives.

HADDOCK WITH A MEDLEY OF VEGETABLES

Serves 2

360g haddock
1 dsp lemon juice
salt and pepper
2 small leeks
90g mushrooms
90g Chinese cabbage
about 7 tbsp water or vegetable stock

Cut the fish into two pieces, sprinkle over the lemon juice and then season. Finely chop the leeks, mushrooms and cabbage. Place 4 tbsp water or vegetable stock in a saucepan, add the leeks, cover, and cook over a gentle heat for 8 minutes, stirring occasionally. Add the mushrooms and cabbage, cover again, and cook gently for 5 minutes. Season to taste. Place the fish on top of the vegetables in the pan. Add another 3 tbsp water or stock, cover and cook for about 5 minutes until the fish is cooked through. Lift out the fish portions and arrange them on two plates, surrounded by the vegetables.

PROVENÇALE CHICKEN KEBABS

Serves 1

  1 x 240g breast of chicken, skin removed
  6 cherry tomatoes
  3 shallots, cut in half
  ½ yellow pepper, cut into 6 pieces
  ½ red pepper, cut into 6 pieces
  1 small courgette
  1 small onion
  2 kebab skewers

Chop the chicken into bite-sized pieces. Onto each kebab skewer, thread half the chicken, 3 cherry tomatoes, 3 halves of shallot, 3 pieces of yellow pepper, 3 pieces of red pepper, 3 pieces of courgette and half the onion, alternating each ingredient along the skewer. Grill until the vegetables are nicely charred and the chicken cooked through. Serve with a Chilled Salad of Mediterranean Vegetables (page 52) on a bed of lettuce.

COD STEAK ON A TRIO OF VEGETABLES

Serves 1

  ½ courgette, sliced
  2ml vegetable stock
  ½ large carrot, sliced
  1 x 180g cod steak
  90ml fish stock
  60ml skimmed milk
  1 bay leaf

Pre-heat the oven to 175°C. Cook the courgette in a little vegetable stock, and in a separate pan do the same with the carrot. Place the cod in an ovenproof dish with the fish stock, skimmed milk and bay leaf. Cover and poach in the oven for 5 minutes until cooked. Whilst the fish is cooking, liquidise the carrot and courgette separately. Place the purées on a plate and lay the fish on top. Serve with some steamed broccoli.

CHICKEN FARCI

Serves 1

1 x 240g chicken breast, skin removed
1 tsp grated carrot
1 tsp chopped shallot
1 tsp chopped tarragon
1 tsp low-fat yoghurt
60ml vegetable stock

To serve

½ red onion, diced
½ green pepper, diced
a small piece of turnip, diced
½ carrot, diced
½ stick celery, diced
1 tsp chopped parsley
2 tsp vegetable stock
a few chives

Pre-heat the oven to 190°C. Remove the small, loose fillet attached to the chicken breast. Chop the chicken finely, and then mix with the grated carrot, chopped shallot, chopped tarragon and yoghurt. Make an incision in the side of the chicken breast without going all the way through. Fill with the stuffing, then seal the cavity with a skewer. Place the chicken in a small ovenproof dish, and then pour the stock around it. Cover with foil, and cook for about 20 minutes, or until the chicken is cooked.

A few minutes before the chicken is ready, cook

the red onion, green pepper, turnip, carrot, celery, parsley and stock in the microwave until soft. Serve the vegetables in the centre of a plate, and then lay the chicken on them. Spoon the chicken cooking juices over the top, and garnish with a few chives.

POSSIBLE RECIPES FOR DAY 7

MINTY CITRUS SALAD

Serves 1

  1 orange
  ½ grapefruit
  1 tbsp low-fat dressing
  1 tsp mint, finely chopped

Peel and segment the fruit, removing all the pith. Arrange alternate segments in a bowl. Mix the dressing with the mint, and pour over.

This recipe can also be used on days 1 and 3

HOT FRUIT SALAD

Serves 2–4

> 120g strawberries
> 120g plums
> 120g cherries
> 60g seedless red grapes
> 2 tbsp orange juice

Pre-heat the oven to 175°C. If the strawberries are large, halve them. Halve and stone the plums and stone the cherries. Place all the ingredients in an ovenproof dish and cook until the juices start to run.

This recipe can also be used on days 1 and 3

RECITE SUGGESTIONS FOR THE WATERCRESS SOUP DIET

ASPARAGUS WITH LEMON DRESSING

Serves 1

> 6 asparagus stalks
> 150ml yoghurt
> rind and juice ½ lemon

Gently scrape the asparagus stalks. Place in a pan of cold water, bring to the boil, and boil for 1 minute. Remove the asparagus and plunge into iced water. When ready to serve, bring the hot water back up to the boil, add the asparagus and boil for about another minute until tender. Mix the yoghurt with the lemon juice, and serve with the asparagus, sprinkled with the zest of the lemon.

NB: This recipe uses nearly half of your daily yoghurt allowance.

This recipe can also be used on days 2, 3 and 6

SOUP DUBARRY

Serves 2

> the white part of 1 small cauliflower
> 375ml vegetable stock
> 250ml skimmed milk
> salt and freshly ground black pepper
> a little grated nutmeg
> a few chives, chopped

Chop the cauliflower into florets and cook in the boiling vegetable stock for 12–15 minutes until tender. Liquidise the cauliflower and stock in a food processor to create a purée. Put the milk in a pan, add the cauliflower purée, season with salt, pepper and a little nutmeg, and heat through. Garnish with the chives and serve.

NB: This recipe uses all of your daily milk allowance.

This recipe can also be used on days 1 and 3

FRENCH BEANS WITH SAVORY

Serves 1

- 240g green beans
- 150ml vegetable stock
- 2 tsp savory, chopped
- 1 dsp low-fat yoghurt
- freshly ground black pepper

Cook the beans in the vegetable stock, drain and transfer to a warm plate. Combine the savory and the yoghurt. Season beans and stock well with black pepper, and top with the yoghurt and savory. Serve immediately.

NB: This recipe uses 1 dsp of your daily yoghurt allowance.

This recipe can also be used on days 1 and 3

RECIPE SUGGESTIONS FOR THE WATERCRESS SOUP DIET

MARINATED VEGETABLES WITH APRICOTS

Serves 1

4 tinned artichoke hearts
240g button mushrooms
2 tbsp lemon juice
1 tsp coriander seeds
1/4 tsp cumin seeds
1 clove garlic
1 apricot, poached in a little water till tender
1 tbsp cider vinegar
a little vegetable stock, if needed
red and white onion rings
fresh coriander leaves, chopped

Drain the tinned artichoke hearts and put them in a large bowl. Trim the base of the mushroom stalks and wipe clean. Bring a saucepan of water to the boil, add 1 tbsp lemon juice and the mushrooms, and cook for 1 minute. Drain the mushrooms and rinse them in cold water. Pat dry and add to the artichokes. Crush the coriander, cumin seeds and garlic in a mortar. Purée the poached apricot in a liquidiser, put in a pan with the crushed mixture and cook for 1 minute. Add the remaining lemon juice and vinegar, and cook for a further minute or two. Add a little stock if needed. Stir this mixture over the mushrooms and artichoke. Cover and chill for about 4 hours. To serve, place the mixture in a salad bowl and garnish with the onion rings and coriander.

This recipe can also be used on Day 3

part 3

keeping weight off – the follow-on diet

As I have already stated, the week-long Watercress Soup Diet must only be used for seven days. After those seven days you will have lost up to ten pounds, and you may go back onto the diet after a four-week break. It is vitally important, however, that you do not just go back to your old eating habits. If you do, you will just put weight straight back on, and you'll never be able to break the cycle.

In this part of the book, you will be helped to

introduce more variety into your meals and to enjoy a less strict routine. You now need to consolidate your new weight and, in the case of those who, despite having lost ten pounds are still overweight, to continue to lose those unwanted pounds. You will gradually be working towards a much healthier and more varied diet that will help you to avoid putting on extra weight.

It cannot be stressed too much that if you want to remain slim, you cannot go back to eating all those foods that have made you the weight you are. Remember too that you can increase the amount of exercise you engage in by moving more purposefully throughout the day. Obvious ways, of course, could be to use the stairs instead of the lift, or to walk to the nearest shop instead of taking the car. Cleaning the house and doing the gardening, if carried out as briskly as possible, will also play their part. In addition, you would benefit by taking some routine exercise two or three times a week. Long walks, swimming, aerobics or working out at the gym will help you to firm up and feel good about yourself. Turn over a new leaf for life!

THE TWO WEEKS FOLLOWING THE DIET

You need to increase your calories quite slowly for the first two weeks, and then gradually move on to a more realistic diet. So for the two weeks following the Watercress Soup Diet, choose from the following. In addition, you are allowed 150ml of skimmed milk and 150ml of very low-fat natural yoghurt. All these recipes serve one person.

A CHOICE OF BREAKFASTS

½ a honeydew melon; 1 large glass unsweetened fruit juice; 1 thin slice (25g) wholemeal bread thinly spread with low-fat spread and topped with Marmite or 15g honey.

Fruit salad composed of ½ mango stoned and sliced, 1 kiwi fruit, 1 peach or nectarine stoned and sliced, and 1 small orange, sliced. Drizzle with 2 tbsp unsweetened orange juice and top with 1 tbsp natural Greek yoghurt.

1 small poached egg served on 1 thin slice (25g) wholemeal bread; 1 large glass unsweetened fruit juice. 25g unsweetened muesli topped with 1 chopped

apple and skimmed or semi-skimmed milk
taken from your allowance.

1 thin slice (25g) wholemeal bread
with low-fat spread;
1 small bunch of grapes.

150ml low-fat fruit yoghurt;
1 large glass unsweetened fruit juice.
2 thin rashers very thinly cut bacon, grilled;
2 grilled cherry tomatoes; 2 grilled mushrooms;
1 thin slice (25g) wholemeal bread;
1 large glass unsweetened fruit juice.

LIGHT LUNCHES

2 Ryvitas or low-calorie crispbreads topped with
cottage cheese and garnished with raw peppers,
celery, tomatoes and/or radish. Serve with a
generous portion of watercress dressed with lemon
juice or low-calorie dressing; 1 orange.

Bowl of watercress soup with 1 thin slice (25g)
wholemeal bread;
1 kiwi fruit.

Mediterranean Salad composed of crisp lettuce,
watercress, tomato, cucumber and raw pepper
slices, about 30g blanched green beans, 1 small
hard-boiled egg and a very small portion of tuna
canned in brine (drained). Drizzle with
1 tsp fat-free dressing or lemon juice; 1 small,
very low-fat yoghurt.

Wholemeal sandwich (no more than 50g of bread) with low-fat spread and filled with thinly sliced chicken or turkey (no skin) and topped with sliced cucumber.

1 medium jacket potato, cooked and the flesh mixed with 1 small carton of cottage cheese and sprinkled with chopped chives. Serve with a watercress salad, dressed with a low-calorie dressing or lemon juice;
2 fresh apricots (or canned in their own juice).

$1/2$ an avocado pear filled with 1 tbsp balsamic vinegar, served on a bed of watercress; 1 apple.

1 thin slice (25g) wholemeal bread, toasted and spread with low-fat spread and topped with 1 small poached egg; watercress and tomato salad;
90g black grapes.

LOW-CALORIE SUPPERS

MARINATED SALMON

1 small salmon fillet marinated with lemon juice
and black pepper, grilled and served with 60g
brown rice combined with cucumber sticks, 1 tbsp
peas and half a red pepper bound together with
1 tbsp low-calorie mayonnaise.

TOMATO AND PEPPER PASTA WITH CRISPY BACON

Make a sauce by heating 1 tbsp olive oil and
sautéing 1 small onion, chopped finely, for 5
minutes. De-seed and finely chop 1 small red
pepper and add to the onion, cook until the
vegetables are soft. If you like garlic add 1 fat
clove, crushed, and cook gently for a further
minute. Add 1 small can of chopped tomatoes and
cook a further 5 or 6 minutes, season with a little
salt and black pepper. Cook 50g wholemeal pasta
in lightly salted water. Drain and top with the
sauce. Grill 25g bacon until crisp, place over the
sauce, and sprinkle over 1 tsp grated Parmesan
cheese. For pudding, 1 peach or nectarine.

HERBY LEMON CHICKEN

Brush a small skinless chicken breast with 1 tsp olive oil, place in an oven dish, pour over 1 tbsp lemon juice and sprinkle with a generous pinch of dried herbs. (You can use fresh herbs – if so, use more.) Cover and cook in a moderate oven for 10 minutes. Uncover and bake a further 5 minutes or until the chicken is quite cooked. Serve with 50g new potatoes, 50g broccoli and 50g sliced carrots. For pudding, a 90g banana.

WATERCRESS OMELETTE

Beat 2 medium eggs with 1 dsp water. Add 1 chopped spring onion and 3 tbsp chopped watercress and season with salt and a little freshly ground black pepper. Heat ½ tbsp olive oil in a non-stick pan and make the omelette in the usual way. Serve with a tomato and basil salad with low-calorie dressing. For pudding, 180g strawberries with a good squeeze of fresh orange juice if desired.

SEAFOOD SALAD

Prepare a salad of green leaves, including
watercress, and top with 150g of seafood such as
prawns, squid, lobster or crab. Sprinkle with lemon
juice and serve with 1 tbsp low-calorie mayonnaise.
For pudding, a bowl of stewed rhubarb sweetened
with low-calorie sweetener and served with 1 tbsp
of low-calorie crème fraîche.

STEAK AND ONIONS

Spray a very little oil on 150g very lean fillet of
steak and grill according to taste. Heat 1 tsp olive
oil in a non-stick pan and sauté one small sliced
onion until cooked and golden brown. Serve with 1
tbsp cooked peas and a grilled tomato garnished
with basil. Follow this with a green salad
containing watercress. For pudding, a 150g serving
of mixed fruit salad dressed with lime juice.

CHICKEN CURRY

Spray a non-stick pan with oil and sauté 1 small
onion until soft. Add a crushed clove of garlic, ½ a
chopped carrot and ½ a stick of chopped celery,

adding a little stock if it is too dry. Now work in 1 tsp curry paste (or more if you prefer a stronger taste) and cook a minute further. Add 1 tsp plain flour and cook for a minute. Take off the heat and add about 175ml chicken stock, a little at a time. Bring to a good simmer. Cut up one skinless chicken thigh and add to the mixture. Cook very slowly until the chicken is cooked, adding more stock as needed. Finish with the juice of $1/2$ a lemon. Serve with 50g brown rice and a watercress salad. For pudding, a large slice of melon.

Good! You have now been watching your weight and eating healthily for three weeks. What you must not do is to return to your old diet. Think about what you eat and how you can cut down on the quantities. Aim for a varied diet and if necessary fill up on extra green and red vegetables and fruit. Eat less cheese and red meat and use less fat in cooking and spreading. Potatoes and pasta are good, but do cut down on the amount that you eat and also consider the fat content of sauces and spreads.

The remainder of this section is intended to put you on the right track for a new, healthy way of eating. You will find fourteen daily menus, complete with recipes. Each recipe contains between 950 and 1500 calories a day. If you stick carefully to this sort of calorific intake, then you will be amazed at the difference in your body. You will be eating healthily, you will not be overindulging, and you will be enjoying your food. You will learn to adjust the amount you regularly eat – and you'll feel better in mind and body for it.

Remember, if you find that you want to shed more weight more quickly, you can always go back on to the Watercress Soup Diet for another week; that's fine as long as you are leaving four weeks between each time you use it.

KEEPING THE WEIGHT OFF – THE FOLLOW-ON DIET

In the following menus, breakfasts, except for Menu 7, are for one portion. Lunch and Dinner menus may be reversed and are for between four and six portions. Some of the lunch recipes given may not be suitable for those who are out at work during the day, so at the end of the chapter you will find some ideas for interesting but low-calorie packed lunches. These recipes may be increased or reduced according to need. If you are catering for people who are not dieting then you must allow for this in the quantity you make. Remember that whatever the quantity of food you make, you must only have a certain fraction of it yourself, in order to stick to your dietary allowance. Thus, if the recipe is for four people, you should only eat a quarter of the food you have made; if it is for six people, you should only permit yourself one-sixth of the total amount. Remember that other people might be able to eat two or even three portions of any given meal, but you must only have one portion. Use your judgement!

MENU 1 – TOTAL CALORIES 1074
ONE BOWL OF WATERCRESS SOUP, PLUS:

BREAKFAST – 193 CALORIES
    100ml fresh orange juice
    1 small egg, boiled or poached
    1 thin slice (25g) wholemeal bread

LUNCH – 346 CALORIES
    Spaghetti with Mushroom Sauce
    1 x 90g apple

DINNER – 535 CALORIES
    Crab Cakes garnished with lemon and
      watercress
    Large green salad with calorie-free dressing
    Stuffed nectarines with a raspberry sauce

SPAGHETTI WITH MUSHROOM SAUCE

Serves 4

1 medium onion, chopped
1 large clove garlic, chopped
2 tbsp virgin olive oil
225g economy mushrooms, cleaned and finely chopped
3 tbsp parsley, chopped
2 small glasses dry white wine
275g spaghetti
150g button mushrooms, cleaned and sliced
150g chestnut mushrooms, cleaned and sliced
salt and freshly ground black pepper
225ml plain yoghurt

Cook the onion and garlic in the oil for 5 minutes over a gentle heat until softened. Bring a pan of lightly salted water to the boil, ready for the pasta.

Add the economy mushrooms to the onions and garlic. Cook gently until the mushrooms soften. Add 2 tbsp of the parsley and the wine, then bring to the boil and simmer for 2-3 minutes until the wine has almost evaporated. Reduce the heat.

Add the spaghetti to the pan of boiling water and cook according to the instructions.

Add the remaining mushrooms to the mixture. Season with salt and pepper. Cover and cook gently for about 5 minutes, until the mushrooms are just tender. Drain the spaghetti and return it to the pan. Stir in the yoghurt. Pour the mushroom mixture onto

the spaghetti and fold in. Divide between four plates
and sprinkle over the remaining parsley.

CRAB CAKES

Serves 4

575g potatoes
115g fresh or canned crab meat (use white and
    brown meat)
2 tbsp fresh chives
juice ½ lemon
1 tsp Worcestershire sauce
3-4 drops chilli sauce
2 eggs (separated)
2 tbsp wholemeal flour
salt and freshly ground black pepper
115g fresh wholemeal breadcrumbs
1 tbsp olive oil

Pre-heat the oven to 220C. Cook the potatoes in
salted boiling water for 10–15 minutes, until tender.
Drain and return to the pan, cooking over a gentle
heat to evaporate as much water as possible. Mash
well and put into a bowl. Add the crab meat, chives,
lemon juice and the chilli sauce and season to taste
with salt. Bind the mixture together with the egg
yolks. Refrigerate the mixture for about an hour
before shaping them into four equal cakes.

Put the seasoned flour and breadcrumbs on
separate flat plates. Lightly whip the egg whites and

mix in ¼ tsp of salt and a good grinding of pepper. Dip the cakes in the flour, then the egg white and finally in the breadcrumbs.

Place the cakes on a non-stick baking tray and sprinkle over the oil. Bake in the oven for about 15 minutes until crisp and golden. Dish up the crab cakes and garnish with the lemon wedges and watercress.

STUFFED NECTARINES WITH A RASPBERRY SAUCE

Serves 4

    180g fresh or frozen raspberries
    sweetener to taste
    2 tbsp chopped nuts
    4 nectarines
    ¼ lemon
    3 tbsp Greek yoghurt (strained)
    3 tbsp low-fat cream or curd cheese
    1 tbsp raisins
    2 tsp clear honey
    sprig of mint

To make the sauce, heat the raspberries gently in a pan, liquidise them and push them through a sieve to remove the seeds. Sweeten if desired and leave to cool. Lightly toast the chopped nuts. (Use a timer or the nuts may burn!) Cut the nectarines in half and remove the stone. Brush the cut edge with lemon juice to prevent discoloration.

Beat the yoghurt into the curd cheese, stir in the cooled nuts, the chopped raisins and the honey. Mix well. Pile the mixture into the nectarines. Divide the sauce between four plates and place two nectarine halves on top. Garnish with a sprig of mint.

MENU 2 – TOTAL CALORIES 938
ONE BOWL OF WATERCRESS SOUP, PLUS:

BREAKFAST – 148 CALORIES
30g unsweetened muesli with 150ml skimmed
    milk
100ml freshly squeezed orange juice

LUNCH – 300 CALORIES
Warm Bacon and Mangetout Salad
Large green salad with watercress
1 medium pear

DINNER – 490 CALORIES
Rice, Chicken and Prawns
Fruits of the Forest

WARM BACON AND MANGETOUT SALAD

Serves 4

50g bread
6 rashers lean back bacon
450g mangetout
1 tbsp lemon juice
1 tbsp chopped herbs
salt and freshly ground black pepper

Heat the oven to 190°C. Remove the crusts from the bread and cut into small cubes. Bake in the oven for about 10 minutes or until golden.

Remove the rind and any fat from the bacon and cut into 15mm strips. Cook in a non-stick frying pan without any fat until golden. Keep warm. Cook the mangetout in lightly salted boiling water until tender but still crisp, about 3-4 minutes, and plunge into ice-cold water for 1 minute to preserve their colour. Plunge the mangetout into boiling water for 5 seconds, just to warm through. Mix the oil and lemon juice in a serving bowl and then add the mangetout (you may like to cut them in half), the bread, bacon and the chopped herbs. Toss well together and serve with the salad.

RICE, CHICKEN AND PRAWNS

Serves 4

4 skinless chicken thighs
2 tbsp olive oil
2 medium onions, chopped
1 large clove garlic, chopped
3 medium tomatoes, skinned,
    de-seeded and diced
1 large red pepper, de-seeded and chopped
570ml chicken stock
1/2 tsp ground turmeric
75g low-fat garlic sausage, chopped
1tsp paprika
225g long-grain brown rice (easy cook)
115g frozen peas
175g peeled prawns
salt and freshly ground black pepper

Fry the chicken in the oil until golden on both sides.
Remove from the heat and put to one side. Reduce
the heat of the pan, add the onions and garlic and
cook gently for 5 minutes. Add the tomatoes and
pepper and cook for a further 2 minutes, stirring
constantly.

Pour the stock into the pan and bring to the boil.
Replace the chicken and cook over a moderate heat
for about 20 minutes.

Add the garlic sausage, paprika, peas and the rice
and stir. Now cook without stirring for about 10
minutes until all the liquid has been absorbed and

the rice is cooked.

Add the peeled prawns to the rice mixture and cook for 2 minutes. Taste and adjust the seasoning before serving.

FRUITS OF THE FOREST

Serves 4

225g blueberries
115g cherries
115g raspberries
115g strawberries
4 heaped tbsp Greek yoghurt
2 tbsp Cassis or Ribena
mint to garnish

Prepare the fruit and arrange on four plates. Divide the yoghurt between the plates and sprinkle with the Cassis or Ribena. Garnish with the mint.

MENU 3 – TOTAL CALORIES 989
ONE BOWL OF WATERCRESS SOUP, PLUS:

BREAKFAST – 293 CALORIES
  1 x 90g banana
  1 thin slice (25g) wholemeal bread
  150ml natural low-fat yoghurt

LUNCH – 314 CALORIES
  2 Ryvita crispbreads
  50g cottage cheese
  50g sliced cucumber
  1 medium tomato
  watercress salad
  1 x 90g apple

DINNER – 382 CALORIES
  Devilled Baked Haddock
  360g frozen peas
  360g new potatoes
  4 medium tomatoes
  Fresh Peach with a Raspberry Coulis

DEVILLED BAKED HADDOCK

Serves 4

4 x 175g haddock fillet
1 medium onion, finely chopped
25g unsalted butter, melted
1 tsp chilli sauce
1 tsp English mustard
1 tsp curry paste
1 tbsp chopped coriander
25g fresh breadcrumbs

Skin the fillets and arrange on a lightly oiled baking tray. Mix the remaining ingredients with the exception of the coriander and spread this mixture evenly over the fillets. Bake in the oven for about 20 minutes. After they have been cooking for 10 minutes, add the halved tomatoes from your dinner allowance to the oven. Serve the fish, sprinkled with the coriander, with the tomatoes and other vegetables

FRESH PEACH WITH A RASPBERRY COULIS

Serves 4

4 ripe peaches
1 tbsp lemon juice
1 tbsp granulated sugar
1 tbsp Ribena
1 tbsp water
225g raspberries (fresh or frozen)
fresh mint

Put the peaches in a large bowl and pour boiling water over them. Allow to stand for 1 minute, then drain and cool. Peel off their skins and sprinkle with the lemon juice to prevent discoloration.

Melt the sugar in a pan with the Ribena and 1 tbsp water before adding the raspberries, and allowing them to soften. Liquidise and then push through a sieve to remove the seeds. Divide the sauce between four plates and place a peach on top. Garnish with the mint. If you prefer you can remove the stones from the peaches and slice them.

MENU 4 – TOTAL CALORIES 1052
ONE BOWL OF WATERCRESS SOUP, PLUS:

BREAKFAST – 211 CALORIES
  200g low-calorie baked beans
  25g wholemeal bread, toasted
  1 tangerine

LUNCH – 256 CALORIES
  90g sardines in brine
  90g lettuce and watercress
  1 medium tomato
  90g fresh black grapes

DINNER – 585 CALORIES
  Spicy Lentils with Lamb and Spinach
  Banana and Raspberry Quickie

SPICY LENTILS WITH LAMB AND SPINACH

Serves 4

75g butter
1 tbsp olive oil
450g lamb, trimmed and cut into 25mm dice
1 large onion, finely sliced
2 large cloves garlic, finely sliced
2 large carrots, sliced into thick batons
400g tin peeled tomatoes
salt and freshly ground black pepper
1 tsp chilli sauce
225g lentils
lamb or vegetable stock
½ tsp cumin powder
½ tsp ground coriander
450g spinach, well washed
2 tbsp chopped parsley

Some lentils need little or no soaking, but if the ones you are using do, it is better to do so overnight.

Heat 50g of the butter with the olive oil in a large, flameproof casserole. Put in the lamb and cook, stirring until it is sealed and golden brown. Remove the lamb with a slotted spoon, leaving any fat behind.

Add the onion, garlic and carrots to the casserole and cook over a moderate heat until softened. Now add the tomatoes, the lamb, the chilli sauce and the lentils. Pour in enough stock to cover. Stir in the spices and simmer for about an hour until the meat and vegetables are tender. You may add a little more stock if the mixture becomes too dry. In the meantime wilt the spinach in the remaining 25g of butter with a little salt. Stir into the casserole and sprinkle with the chopped parsley.

BANANA AND RASPBERRY QUICKIE

Serves 4

   1 large banana
   225g frozen raspberries
   mint to garnish

Put the banana and the unthawed frozen raspberries into a blender and process for 2–3 minutes, until you have a smooth purée. Spoon into four small dishes and serve at once garnished with the mint.

MENU 5 – 1033 CALORIES
ONE BOWL OF WATERCRESS SOUP, PLUS:

BREAKFAST - 166 CALORIES
    180g porridge (as cooked)
    Sweetener or salt for the porridge
    90g strawberries

LUNCH – 373 CALORIES
    270g jacket potato
    50g cottage cheese with chopped chives
    Stewed rhubarb sweetened with sweetener

DINNER – 494 CALORIES
    Chicken with Pasta and Tinned Artichoke Hearts
    Mixed salad
    Bramley Apple with Currants

CHICKEN WITH PASTA AND TINNED ARTICHOKE HEARTS

Serves 4

2 tbsp extra virgin olive oil
2 tbsp white wine vinegar
1 large onion, finely chopped
2 large uncooked skinless chicken breasts,
   cut into 50mm strips
2 glasses white wine
juice of 1 lemon
400g tinned artichoke hearts,
   drained and cut into bite-sized pieces
1 tbsp fresh tarragon, chopped, or 1 tsp dried
350g tagliatelle verdi
75g small mangetout (or cut them in half)
115g broccoli, broken into florets
4 tbsp strained Greek yoghurt
salt and freshly ground black pepper

Heat the oil in a frying pan, add the vinegar and onion and cook for 3 minutes over a medium heat. Add the chicken and cook for a further 3 minutes, stirring occasionally. Add the wine and the lemon juice and reduce the heat so that the sauce is just simmering. Add the artichokes and tarragon to the chicken. Stir in the yoghurt, adjust the seasoning and continue to simmer over a low heat.

Cook the pasta in a large pan of boiling salted water. Cook the broccoli florets and mangetout in a smaller pan of boiling salted water for 2 or 3 minutes.

Drain the pasta and vegetables as soon as they are cooked. Spoon the chicken, artichokes and sauce over the pasta. Divide between four plates and arrange the green vegetables around the edge of the plates.

BRAMLEY APPLE WITH CURRANTS

Serves 1

1x85g apple
25g currants
sweetener to taste
apple juice

Core the apple and stuff with the currants and some sweetener to taste. Moisten with a little apple juice and either bake in the oven or in the microwave until cooked. Try not to let it collapse!

MENU 6 – 1050
ONE BOWL OF WATERCRESS SOUP, PLUS:

BREAKFAST – 265 CALORIES
  2 thin slices (50g) wholemeal bread
  15g low-fat spread
  60g smoked salmon

LUNCH – 270 CALORIES
  Apple and Parsnip Soup
  1 thin slice (25g) wholemeal bread
  Fruit salad made from 90g orange, 90g melon and
  90g strawberries

DINNER – 515 CALORIES
  Monkfish with Three Vegetables
  Bread and Butter Pudding

APPLE AND PARSNIP SOUP

Serves 6

1 medium onion, finely chopped
2 tbsp olive oil
a good grinding of nutmeg
450g parsnips, peeled and roughly chopped
250g Cox's apples, peeled,
  cored and roughly chopped
225ml semi-skimmed milk
850ml vegetable stock
salt and freshly ground black pepper
chopped parsley to garnish

Sauté the onions in the oil until transparent. Stir in the nutmeg and add the parsnips, apple, milk and stock. Bring to the boil, then reduce the heat and simmer for about 20 minutes until the parsnips are tender. Allow to cool slightly. Pour the soup into a blender or food processor and blend until smooth. Garnish with the parsley.

MONKFISH WITH THREE VEGETABLES

Serves 4

450g monkfish tails
salt and 1 tbsp coarsely crushed black
  peppercorns
1 tbsp extra virgin olive oil
15g unsalted butter
150ml fish stock
1 tsp arrowroot
4 tbsp single cream
2 tbsp brandy
3 carrots, peeled and cut into ribbons
3 courgettes, washed and cut into ribbons
watercress

Skin the tails and remove the pink membranes. Cut down either side of the central bone to remove the fillets. Gently rub a little salt and the crushed peppercorns into the fish and fry for about 10 minutes in the oil and butter, turning until well sealed. Add the fish stock and simmer gently for about 10 minutes. Remove the fish.

Mix the arrowroot with a little water to make a paste and stir into the sauce. Add the cream and the brandy and stir for a few minutes until slightly thickened. Replace the fish.

Cook the vegetables in a little lightly salted water until tender. Serve the fish garnished with the vegetables and watercress.

BREAD AND BUTTER PUDDING

Serves 4

4 thin slices white bread
50g butter
115g currants
2 eggs and 1 extra yolk
285ml semi-skimmed milk
rind of ½ lemon
1 tsp vanilla extract
2 tbsp runny honey
¼ tsp freshly ground nutmeg

Butter the slices of bread and cut each slice into four triangles. Grease a 570ml pie dish and arrange the bread in layers, sprinkling each with currants. Make sure that the final layer is butter-side up.

Beat the eggs together and add the milk. Stir in the lemon rind and the vanilla extract. Pour the liquid over the bread and drizzle the honey over the mixture. Leave to stand for about 1 hour. Heat the oven to 180°C.

Sprinkle the top of the pudding with the nutmeg and bake for about 30 minutes or until well risen and golden brown. Serve immediately.

MENU 7 – TOTAL CALORIES 1127

ONE BOWL OF WATERCRESS SOUP, PLUS:

BREAKFAST – 381 CALORIES
  Smoked Haddock Kedgeree
  200ml fresh orange juice

LUNCH – 234 CALORIES
  Carrot and Tomato Soup with Cardamom
  1 thin slice (25g) wholemeal bread
  1 x 90g banana

DINNER – 512 CALORIES
  Oriental Beef and Vegetables
  350g brown rice
  Green salad dressed with lemon juice
  180g strawberries moistened with fresh
    orange juice

SMOKED HADDOCK KEDGEREE

Serves 6

3 eggs
2 tbsp groundnut oil
1 green pepper, de-seeded and chopped
3 sticks celery, trimmed and chopped small
1 small onion, finely chopped
2 tsp curry powder
¼ tsp cayenne pepper
350g basmati rice
850ml fish or vegetable stock
salt and freshly ground black pepper
350g smoked haddock
285ml semi-skimmed milk
2 tbsp freshly chopped parsley

Hard-boil the eggs and put immediately into very cold running water. Keep on one side in their shells. Rinse the rice well and leave to drain in a colander.

Heat the oil in a large pan, add the chopped vegetables and cook over a moderate heat for 10-15 minutes, stirring frequently until softened. Add the curry powder and cayenne pepper and stir constantly for a further 2 minutes. Stir in the rice, followed by the hot stock. Bring to the boil stirring constantly. Lower the heat and season with salt and pepper. Be careful not to add too much, as the fish is quite salty. Cover and simmer for 15 minutes, until the rice is tender and almost all the stock has been absorbed.

Shell the eggs and put to one side. Put the fish, skin-side down, in a single layer in a frying pan and pour over the milk and enough water to just cover. Season with pepper to taste and bring to the boil. Lower the heat. Remove the fish and flake it, removing the skin and bones.

Gently fold the fish into the rice together with the parsley. Transfer to a serving dish. Cut the hard-boiled eggs into quarters and use to garnish the kedgeree. Serve immediately.

CARROT AND TOMATO SOUP WITH CARDAMOM

Serves 4

9 fresh green or white cardamom pods
  (do not use ground)
1 onion, finely chopped
1½ tbsp olive oil
275g carrots, trimmed and roughly chopped
275g fresh tomatoes, skinned,
  de-seeded and chopped
975ml vegetable stock
salt and freshly ground black pepper
chopped coriander for garnish

Crush the pods and place seeds and pods in a piece of muslin and tie securely. Sauté the onion in the oil in a large pan until transparent. Add the carrots and tomatoes and stir for 3 minutes. Add the stock and cardamom pods and bring to the boil. Reduce the heat and simmer for about 30 minutes until the carrots are tender. Remove the pods from the soup and allow to cool before squeezing the bag into the soup in order to extract all the flavour.

Purée the vegetables and their liquid in a blender and when ready to serve, heat gently and sprinkle with the garnish.

ORIENTAL BEEF AND VEGETABLES

Serves 4

    8 x 50g slices entrecôte steak
    50g leeks
    50g carrots
    50g green beans
    50g young turnips
    8 small shallots
    4 tsp vegetable oil
    1 tbsp red wine vinegar
    385ml red wine
    150ml beef stock
    1 tbsp oyster sauce
    1 tbsp soy sauce
    1 ½ tsp arrowroot or cornflour
    1 tbsp water

Trim all fat from the beef, and bat well with a rolling pin until quite thin. Cut all the vegetables, except the shallots, into thin strips. Plunge them into boiling water for 30 seconds to blanch and then drain.

Put the slices of beef on individual pieces of clingfilm and divide the vegetables over them. Now roll up each slice tightly in the clingfilm and screw up the overlapping film at the sides to tighten even further. When you release the rolls from the clingfilm they should have stuck well together.

Heat 1 tbsp of the oil in a large frying pan over a medium heat and brown the beef rolls on all sides for about 5 minutes. Remove from the pan. Cut the shallots into thin rings. Add the remaining oil and the vinegar to the pan and sauté the shallots for about 5 minutes until they are transparent and the vinegar is reduced. Add the wine, stock, oyster sauce and soy sauce and bring to a simmer. Mix the arrowroot or cornflour with 1 tbsp water, stirring into the sauce until thickened.

Return the beef rolls to the pan and simmer for 5 minutes. Remove to individual plates and cover with the sauce. Serve with boiled rice and green salad.

MENU 8 – TOTAL CALORIES 1017

ONE BOWL OF WATERCRESS SOUP, PLUS:

BREAKFAST – 138 CALORIES
   ½ grapefruit
   2 thin slices (50g) wholemeal bread
   15g honey

LUNCH – 455 CALORIES
   Egg and Stir-Fry Vegetables with Oyster Sauce
   150ml low-fat fruit yoghurt

DINNER – 424 CALORIES
   Spicy Chicken with Dried Fruits
   Colourful Veggies
   25g cottage cheese
   1 water biscuit

EGG AND STIR-FRY VEGETABLES WITH OYSTER SAUCE

Serves 4

2 tbsp vegetable oil
2 tbsp sesame seed oil
2 large cloves garlic, finely chopped
225g broccoli florets
1 red pepper, de-seeded and cut into strips
225g green beans, trimmed and cut in three
2 carrots, peeled and sliced into rounds
50g spring onions, sliced
3 tbsp oyster sauce
1 small green chilli
175g bean sprouts
1 tbsp light soy sauce
1 tbsp caster sugar
juice of 1 lime
salt and freshly ground black pepper
1 hard-boiled egg to garnish

Heat the vegetable oil and the sesame seed oil in a wok or large frying pan. Add the garlic and stir over gentle heat for about 1 minute. Stir in all the remaining vegetables except the bean sprouts and add the oyster sauce. Stir-fry for about 4 minutes.

Add the remaining ingredients and stir-fry for another 2 minutes. Sprinkle the lime juice over the vegetables, season and serve garnished with the chopped hard-boiled egg.

SPICY CHICKEN WITH DRIED FRUITS

Serves 4

285ml chicken stock
150ml fresh orange juice
2 tsp paprika
2 tsp ground ginger
1/2 tsp ground cinnamon
1/4 tsp ground allspice
250g ready-to-eat dried fruit salad
1 kilo skinless bone-in chicken thighs
salt and freshly ground black pepper

Pour the chicken stock and the orange juice into a flameproof casserole dish, then add the spices and stir well. Add the dried fruit and bring slowly to the boil, stirring continuously. Add the chicken and season to taste. Baste the chicken well with the liquid.

Lower the heat and cover the pan with a tightly fitting lid. Simmer very gently for about 30 minutes, until the chicken is tender. Lift the lid occasionally during cooking, and stir to ensure even cooking. Adjust the seasoning.

COLOURFUL VEGGIES

Serves 4

40g butter
3 tbsp water
4 leeks, washed and thinly sliced
1 tbsp extra virgin olive oil
2 yellow peppers, de-seeded and sliced into
    strips
1 red pepper, de-seeded and sliced into strips
1½ tbsp fresh mixed herbs
salt and freshly ground black pepper

Melt the butter in a pan with 3 tbsp water and add the leeks with a little salt. Cover the pan and cook over a medium heat for 8 minutes until tender.

Uncover the pan, add the oil and raise the heat. Sauté the peppers for 2 minutes. Add a little more water, lower the heat and cook for a further 2 minutes until the peppers are soft and there is a sweet sauce in the pan. Add the herbs, season and serve.

MENU 9 – TOTAL CALORIES 1015
ONE BOWL OF WATERCRESS SOUP, PLUS:

BREAKFAST – 235 CALORIES
    ½ grapefruit
    25g lean lightly cured bacon, grilled
    240g grilled tomatoes
    1 thin slice (25g) wholemeal bread

LUNCH – 330 CALORIES
    Spicy Lentil Soup
    1 medium orange

DINNER 450 CALORIES
    Plaice with Watercress Sauce
    120g boiled potatoes
    green salad
    1 medium orange

SPICY LENTIL SOUP

Serves 4

115g red lentils
1 tbsp extra virgin olive oil
1 tsp cumin powder
2 tsp coriander powder
1 tsp turmeric
1 dried red chilli
50g carrots, finely diced
115g potatoes, finely diced
1 onion, finely diced
1.1l vegetable stock
salt and freshly ground black pepper
chopped parsley to garnish

Wash the lentils and drain. Heat the oil in a large pan and cook the onion until transparent. Add the spices and cook for 2 minutes, stirring continuously.

Put the carrots and potatoes in the saucepan with the lentils and stock. Bring to the boil, reduce the heat and simmer for 1 hour until tender.

Season to taste and serve sprinkled with the chopped parsley.

PLAICE WITH WATERCRESS SAUCE

Serves 4

- 1 small onion, finely chopped
- 15g butter
- 1 bunch watercress (or 1 large pack)
- 5 tbsp single cream
- 25g soft low-fat cheese
- 8 small fillets of plaice
- 2 tbsp vegetable oil
- salt and freshly ground black pepper
- watercress sprigs to garnish
- 1 lemon

Gently sauté the onion in the butter for 5 minutes. Add the watercress and cook for a further 2 minutes until the watercress is wilted without losing its colour. Blend this mixture in a food processor and while the motor is running, add the cream and the cheese. Blend until smooth.

Brush the plaice fillets lightly with oil and place on a lightly oiled baking tray. Season to taste and grill until lightly golden.

Re-heat the sauce gently and divide between four plates. Dish the fish at the side and garnish with sprigs of watercress and a quarter of a lemon.

MENU 10 – TOTAL CALORIES 943
ONE BOWL OF WATERCRESS SOUP, PLUS:

BREAKFAST – 228 CALORIES
90g banana
150ml very low-fat yoghurt
1 thin slice (25g) wholemeal bread

LUNCH – 255 CALORIES
Greek Salad with Feta
1 thin slice (25g) wholemeal bread
Stewed rhubarb with sweetener served with 60g
low-fat ice cream

DINNER – 460 CALORIES
Green Tagliatelle with Chicken and Artichoke
Hearts
Mixed green salad with cucumber
Fresh Fruit Salad with Stem Ginger

GREEK SALAD WITH FETA

Serves 4

- 2 large red peppers
- 2 large yellow peppers
- 4 spring onions
- 2 tbsp extra virgin olive oil
- 1 tbsp white wine vinegar
- 1 large oak leaf lettuce
- 175g feta cheese
- fresh basil leaves
- 1 tsp toasted sesame seeds
- salt and freshly ground black pepper

Grill the peppers until the skins have blackened. Seal in a plastic bag until cool, when the skins should come off quite easily.

To create a dressing, trim the spring onions and thinly slice both the bulb and the green part. Whisk together the oil and the vinegar and add the spring onions and season to taste.

Prepare the lettuce and divide between four plates. Skin and de-seed the peppers and cut into thin strips. Put them onto the lettuce and pour over the dressing. Crumble the cheese over the top and sprinkle the sesame seeds on too; season with pepper and garnish with the torn basil leaves.

GREEN TAGLIATELLE WITH CHICKEN AND ARTICHOKE HEARTS

Serves 4

2 tbsp olive oil
1 large onion, finely chopped
2 tbsp sherry vinegar
2 raw skinless chicken breasts, sliced into
    chunky strips
2 glasses dry white wine
juice of 1 lemon
1 tbsp fresh tarragon, roughly chopped
400g tinned artichoke hearts, drained and cut
    into bite-sized pieces
4 tbsp Greek yoghurt
350g green tagliatelle
75g mangetout, trimmed and halved
115g broccoli florets
salt and freshly ground black pepper

Heat 2 tbsp of the oil in a pan and add the onion and the vinegar. Cook over a medium heat for about 3 minutes. Add the chicken and cook for another 3 minutes, stirring from time to time. Add the wine and the lemon juice and reduce the heat to a simmer.

Add the chopped tarragon leaves to the chicken together with the artichokes. Stir in the yoghurt, adjust the seasoning and continue to simmer over a low heat.

Cook the pasta in a large pan according to the

instructions. Cook the mangetout and broccoli in boiling water for a few minutes. Drain the pasta and the vegetables. Spoon the chicken, artichokes and sauce on top of the pasta and arrange the vegetables around the dish.

FRESH FRUIT SALAD WITH STEM GINGER

Serves 6

 50g caster sugar
 1 tbsp water
 1 tbsp Cointreau or other liqueur
 1 small pineapple
 1 Ogen melon
 2 ripe comice pears
 juice of ½ lemon
 50g stem ginger
 fresh mint to garnish (ginger mint would be
    especially tasty)

Place the sugar in a basin with 1 tbsp water and bring very slowly to the boil. The sugar needs to dissolve before the water boils. Simmer until the liquid is clear and then add the liqueur. Put to one side.

Cut away the outer skin of the pineapple and slice the flesh into small pieces. Cut the melon into four and remove the skin and the seeds. Cut up in the same way as the pineapple. Peel, core and cut the pears into uniform slices. Sprinkle the pear slices with the lemon juice to retain their colour. Finely slice the ginger. Mix all the fruits and the ginger together and mix with the cooled syrup of sugar and liqueur. Cover with film and chill for 1 hour if possible. Garnish with the mint.

MENU 11 – TOTAL CALORIES 1053
ONE BOWL OF WATERCRESS SOUP, PLUS:

BREAKFAST 246 CALORIES
    2 grilled tomatoes
    100g reduced-calorie baked beans
    25g wholemeal bread
    200ml fresh orange juice

LUNCH – 270 CALORIES
    Italian Hard-Boiled Eggs
    large watercress salad dressed with lemon juice
    1 pear

DINNER – 537 CALORIES
    Ham and Pea Risotto
    90g kiwi fruit dressed with lime juice

ITALIAN HARD-BOILED EGGS

Serves 4

4 eggs
1 clove garlic
2 large sprigs of basil
25g pine nuts
25g grated Parmesan cheese
1 tbsp virgin olive oil
freshly ground black pepper
2 very large tomatoes
extra basil to garnish

Hard-boil the eggs and cool them under cold running water. Remove the shells and cut in half lengthways. Remove the yolks.

Crush the garlic and place in a liquidiser together with the basil sprigs and pine nuts. Blend until smooth. Add the egg yolks and the Parmesan and blend again. Pour in the olive oil and blend once more. Season to taste using plenty of black pepper. Pile the mixture into the egg whites. Slice up the tomatoes and divide between four plates. Place the stuffed eggs on top and garnish with the basil.

HAM AND PEA RISOTTO

Serves 4

4 thin slices lean cooked ham
2 tbsp olive oil
15g butter
1 medium onion, finely chopped
350g short grain risotto rice
150ml dry white wine
1.1l vegetable stock
75g frozen peas
salt and freshly ground black pepper
50g freshly grated Parmesan cheese

Remove any fat from the ham and cut into strips. Heat the oil and butter over a gentle heat and cook the onion until it is soft and golden. Add the rice to the onions and cook over a moderate heat for 5 minutes until the grains begin to burst. Heat the stock.

Stir the wine into the rice and cook until it has been absorbed. Add 150ml of the hot stock. Mix well and continue cooking over a moderate heat until absorbed, stirring continuously.

Continue cooking for a further 20 minutes adding the stock 150ml at a time until the rice is tender and the texture is creamy. Add the peas with the last measure of stock and season to taste. Fold in the ham and 25g of the Parmesan. Divide the risotto between four bowls and sprinkle on the remaining Parmesan.

MENU 12 – TOTAL CALORIES – 1055
ONE BOWL OF WATERCRESS SOUP, PLUS:

BREAKFAST – 225 CALORIES
   2 thin slices (50g) wholemeal bread with low-fat
      spread and Marmite
   150ml tomato juice

LUNCH – 270 CALORIES
   Watercress, Apple and Parmesan Cheese Salad
   150g fresh or frozen raspberries

DINNER – 560 CALORIES
   Lean Irish Stew
   150g steamed broccoli per serving
   Gooseberry Fool

WATERCRESS, APPLE AND PARMESAN CHEESE SALAD

Serves 4

175g watercress
115g Parmesan, sliced into large shavings
2 tbsp extra virgin olive oil
juice of ½ orange
2 tsp white wine vinegar
1 tsp Dijon mustard
½ tsp horseradish sauce
2 Cox's apples
salt and freshly ground black pepper

Wash and prepare the salad, removing any long stems. Dry in a salad spinner or with kitchen paper. Mix together the oil, orange juice, vinegar, mustard and horseradish in a bowl and season to taste with salt and pepper. Wash, but do not peel the apple. Cut into four and remove the core. Now cut it into 15mm cubes. Mix the apple with the salad and mix well with the dressing. Scatter the Parmesan over the mixture.

THE WATERCRESS SOUP DIET

122

LEAN IRISH STEW

Serves 4

    450g lean neck of lamb fillet
    900g potatoes, peeled and thinly sliced
    2 large onions, sliced into rings
    2 tsp fresh chopped rosemary, or 1 tsp dried
    2 tsp fresh chopped thyme, or 1 tsp dried
    salt and freshly ground black pepper
    lamb stock
    chopped parsley to garnish

Pre-heat the oven to 180°C. Cut the meat into thin slices, trimming away any fat. Line the bottom of a casserole dish with a layer of potatoes, then a layer of onion rings and a layer of lamb. Sprinkle with a little rosemary and thyme and season. Continue layering the meat, vegetables and herbs, finishing with a layer of potato.

Pour in enough stock to half fill the casserole dish and slowly bring to the boil. Cover with foil and the casserole lid and cook in the oven for about 2½ hours until the potatoes and lamb are tender. Uncover the casserole for the last 20 minutes of cooking to brown the potatoes.

Garnish with the chopped parsley. Serve with about 150g of steamed broccoli.

MENU 13 – 1030 CALORIES
ONE BOWL OF WATERCRESS SOUP, PLUS:

BREAKFAST – 222 CALORIES
  240g grilled tomatoes
  1 thin slice (25g) wholemeal bread
  15g low-fat spread
  150ml apple juice

LUNCH – 225 CALORIES
  Omelette made with 2 small eggs and 12g of
    mature low-fat Cheddar cheese. Make your
    omelette in a non-stick pan with just a light
    spray of oil.
  1 wholemeal biscuit

DINNER – 583 CALORIES
  Sirloin Steak with Mustard and Peppercorn
    Sauce
  90g carrots per serving
  180g cauliflower per serving
  Fresh Fruit Jelly with Cointreau

SIRLOIN STEAK WITH MUSTARD AND PEPPERCORN SAUCE

Serves 4

4 x 175g sirloin steaks
2 shallots, finely chopped
2 cloves garlic, finely chopped
1 tsp green peppercorns, crushed
2 tsp coarse grain mustard
2 tbsp brandy
225ml Greek yoghurt
juice of ½ lemon
salt and freshly ground black pepper

Trim the steaks of any fat. Make a griddle or heavy frying pan very hot and spray with a little oil. Fry the steaks in the hot pan for 2 minutes on each side. Reduce the heat and cook for up to 2-3 minutes more. Eight minutes will give a well-done steak; reduce the cooking time by half for a rare steak. Keep warm.

Add the shallots and garlic to the pan juices. Cook over a low heat, stirring until lightly coloured. Add the crushed peppercorns, mustard and brandy. Stir in the yoghurt and lemon juice. Heat gently without boiling and pour over the steaks. Serve with the vegetables.

FRESH FRUIT JELLY WITH COINTREAU

Serves 4

6 large oranges
340ml water
115g sugar
powdered gelatine
2 tbsp Cointreau

Squeeze the juice from 5 of the oranges and add 340ml of water. Measure the quantity of liquid in order to assess how much gelatine you will need. The recommended amounts will be on the packet. Thinly pare the zest from the remaining orange. Put the juice, water and sugar together with the zest in a large pan and bring slowly to the boil making sure that the sugar dissolves. Dissolve the gelatine as per the packet instructions. Remove the zest from the large pan. Reduce the heat and stir in the gelatine and simmer until the gelatine is completely incorporated.

Strain the jelly liquid into a wet mould and stir in the liqueur. Leave in the refrigerator to set for about 2 hours. When set, dip the mould into hot water and upturn on a suitable plate. Decorate the base of the jelly with segments cut from the remaining orange. Scatter the thinly cut zest over the top.

MENU 14 – 1023 CALORIES
ONE BOWL OF WATERCRESS SOUP, PLUS:

BREAKFAST – 165 CALORIES
   120g tinned prunes
   1 thin slice (25g) wholemeal bread
   15g low-fat spread
   15g marmalade

LUNCH – 231 CALORIES
   Mediterranean Pasta
   90g black grapes

DINNER – 627 CALORIES
   Irish Braised Beef
   90g mashed potatoes per serving sprinkled with
      chopped chives
   90g steamed cabbage per serving
   Rosy Poached Pears

MEDITERRANEAN PASTA

Serves 4

2 tbsp virgin olive oil
1 medium onion, thinly sliced
1 red pepper, de-seeded and cut into thin strips
1 yellow pepper, de-seeded and cut into thin
    strips
2 medium courgettes, cut into thin strips
1 small aubergine, peeled and cut into thin strips
2 cloves garlic, crushed
450g tinned chopped tomatoes
1 tbsp tomato purée
2 tsp chopped fresh basil
1tsp dried herbes de Provence
salt and freshly ground black pepper
1 glass red wine
275g fusilli pasta
75g Parmesan cheese, grated

Heat the oil in a heavy saucepan or casserole dish.
Add the sliced onion and cook over a gentle heat for
about 5 minutes, stirring frequently until soft. Add
the peppers and cook for a further 5 minutes,
stirring frequently. Add the courgettes, aubergine
and garlic and continue to cook for a few more
minutes. Now add the tomatoes, tomato purée and
herbs. Season to taste.

Bring to the boil, stirring often. Then lower the
heat, half cover the pan and simmer for 20 minutes.
Stir occasionally and add a little water or wine if the

sauce seems dry. Warm a large serving bowl.

Cook the pasta according to the instructions. Drain, and turn into the warmed bowl. Pour the sauce over the pasta and toss well. Garnish with the Parmesan.

IRISH BRAISED BEEF

Serves 4

700g braising steak, cut into 40mm cubes
2 large onions, quartered
115g button mushrooms
4 large carrots, cut crossways into 4
4 sticks celery, cut crossways into 4
½ tsp dried mixed herbs
1 bay leaf
1 tbsp tomato purée
1tsp brown sugar
570ml beef stock
285ml Guinness
1 tbsp cornflour
1 tbsp water
salt and freshly ground black pepper
chopped parsley to garnish

Pre-heat the oven to 160°C. Place the meat and vegetables in an ovenproof casserole along with the mixed herbs, bay leaf, tomato purée, sugar, beef stock and Guinness. Stir to mix thoroughly. Gently bring the stew to the boil, then cover and transfer to the oven. Cook very gently in the oven for about 2¹/₂ hours until the meat is quite tender.

Remove the meat. Mix the cornflour with 1 tbsp water until smooth, then stir into the casserole. Bring to the boil, stirring until thickened. Adjust seasoning to taste. Return the meat to the casserole and warm gently through. Transfer to a serving dish, garnish with freshly chopped parsley and serve with the vegetables.

ROSY POACHED PEARS

Serves 4

4 firm dessert pears
285ml red wine
¹/₂ glass Cassis (optional)
1¹/₂ tbsp lemon juice
1 cinnamon stick or 2 tsp ground cinnamon
115g caster sugar
1tsp ground ginger
1 tbsp runny honey
6 cloves
4 bay leaves
a twist of freshly ground black pepper
mint sprigs to garnish

Peel the pears and leave them whole with their stalks on. Pour the red wine and optional Cassis into a large pan and add the lemon juice, cinnamon, sugar, ginger, honey, cloves, bay leaves and black pepper. Heat gently, stirring until the sugar has dissolved.

Add the pears, spoon the mixture over them and cover the pan. Reduce to a low heat and – keeping the liquid just below boiling point – poach gently for about 1 hour, turning occasionally until the pears are soft but still whole. The time they take will be determined by the ripeness of the pears.

Remove the pears from the liquid and arrange on a serving dish or individual plates. Strain the liquid through a sieve and discard the spices. Reduce the sauce until there is just enough to cover the pears. Coat the pears with the sauce, cover and chill. Garnish with the mint sprigs.

The lunch recipes in this section may not be convenient for those who have to take their midday meal away from home. It is possible to buy prepared sandwiches that are low in calories, but if you prefer to take your own packed lunch, here are some ideas to inspire you. In each case, 2 x 25g wholemeal bread slices and 25g low-fat spread are used:

60g smoked salmon on 25g cottage cheese; a 90g apple (340 calories)

Celery, 90g apple, and 12g walnuts; a 90g orange (326 calories)

90g cold chicken, watercress; a 90g banana (327 calories)
25g cheddar cheese, 90g tomato; a 90g kiwi fruit (391 calories)

1 egg, cress; 150ml low-fat natural yoghurt (359 calories)

50g prawns covered with sliced cucumber; 1 pear (280 calories)

part 4

entertaining on the diet

Now that you look great and feel better about yourself, it is time to do a little showing off – and what better way than to invite a few friends round? This section gives you six great dinner party recipes, all of which are perfect for entertaining without deviating from your new regime. If your friends are also trying to lose weight they will appreciate delicious low-calorie food. And if they are not weight-watching, they will never know, because these recipes are so scrumptious!

ENTERTAINING ON THE DIET

When entertaining, be careful to eat frugally at breakfast and lunch (a bowl of hot watercress soup and a piece of fruit would be an ideal lunch – and a tasty one too!) to save your calories for the dinner party, and remember that though you might make extra food to enable your guests to have extra helpings, this does not apply to you. Eat slowly and savour every mouthful. You will have noticed also that fats, oils and cream have been used in the recipes, but in small amounts. By now you will have discovered that food does not have to be rich to be delicious, so just because you are entertaining, don't be tempted to add extra butter and cream.

You will see that some of these menus are higher in calories than those you have been using just lately, but it is assumed that you won't be preparing such meals very often. In any case, you must be careful to eat less on these occasions – you will know by now how much you can eat without putting on weight.

DINNER PARTY 1

(FOR 4 PEOPLE) – 770 CALORIES

ENTERTAINING ON THE DIET

STARTER – MEDITERRANEAN GRILLED VEGETABLES

For the Marinade

2 tbsp extra virgin olive oil
1 tbsp balsamic vinegar
freshly ground back pepper
a little freshly ground sea salt
15g runny honey
1 tbsp fresh lemon juice

8 trimmed asparagus spears
2 medium red onions, cut in half lengthways
2 medium red peppers, cored, de-seeded and cut in
   half lengthways
2 medium aubergines, sliced
4 medium courgettes, cut lengthways into batons
12 cherry tomatoes
2 tbsp of fresh oregano or marjoram, chopped
2 tbsp of fresh basil, chopped
2 tbsp fresh parsley, chopped
430g canned kidney beans, drained and rinsed.

Mix and reserve the ingredients for the marinade.

Char the peppers under the grill, and peel. Blanch the asparagus for 2 minutes and the onions for 3 minutes. Drain well and dry thoroughly. Place together with the other vegetables under a hot grill until they are soft and slightly charred. Place in a bowl.

Add the herbs and kidney beans to the bowl. Pour over the marinade and mix well, turning gently. Leave to marinate for 1–2 hours. Serve with crusty bread.

MAIN COURSE – PASTA WITH SALMON AND VEGETABLES

225g fresh broccoli
275g pasta (penne would be a good choice)
225g fresh salmon
150ml dry white wine
6 good-sized sprigs of fresh tarragon
175g low-fat fromage frais
4 tbsp whipping cream
3 tsp lemon juice
salt and freshly ground pepper
lemon wedges and watercress for garnish

Prepare the broccoli by cutting up into bite-size florets. Cut the stalks into very small cubes. Cook the pasta in boiling salted water for 10 minutes, then add the broccoli and cook for a further 2 minutes.

Whilst the pasta is boiling, remove any skin and bones from the salmon and dice into 25mm cubes. Put the fish into a large pan with a pinch of salt, the wine and enough water to cover. Bring gently to the boil and simmer for 3 minutes. Remove with a slotted spoon, cover and keep warm.

Remove the leaves from four of the tarragon stalks, chop them finely and combine with the fromage frais and single cream. Stir into the fish juices remaining in the pan and heat very gently until just warmed. Drain the pasta and broccoli in a colander. Reserve a few of the florets for garnish and add the rest of the broccoli and pasta to the tarragon sauce. Stir in the lemon juice, season to taste, and re-heat gently for 2 or 3 minutes.

Spoon the pasta onto warm plates and arrange the salmon over the top. Garnish with the broccoli florets, sprigs of tarragon and lemon wedges. Serve immediately.

DESSERT – SUMMER FRUIT BRÛLÉ

100g blueberries or blackberries
100g raspberries
125g strawberries, hulled and sliced
115g redcurrants or blackcurrants
low-calorie sweetener to taste
360g natural low-fat fromage frais
100g demerara sugar

Mix together all the fruit and divide between four ramekin dishes. Sprinkle a little sweetener over the fruit if desired. Spoon the fromage frais over the fruit, smoothing it out to completely cover the surface. Chill for 10 minutes.

Pre-heat the grill and place the desserts on a baking sheet and sprinkle the sugar over the top. Grill until the sugar melts and bubbles – or use a blow-torch to achieve the same effect. Chill thoroughly before serving

Did you know...?
According to Greek legend, Zeus, the father of the gods, is said to have eaten watercress to strengthen himself against his murderous father, Cronos.

DINNER PARTY 2

(FOR 4 PEOPLE) – 985 CALORIES

STARTER – RIPE PEARS WITH ROQUEFORT CHEESE

75g Roquefort cheese
75g very low-fat soft cheese
150ml natural low-fat yoghurt
cayenne pepper
50g shelled walnuts
1 tbsp chopped fresh tarragon
½ lemon
1 tsp tarragon vinegar
4 ripe comice pears
8 sprigs watercress.
tarragon leaves to garnish

Using a fork, mash the Roquefort together with the soft cheese, 1 tbsp of the yoghurt and the cayenne pepper. Divide between two bowls. Reserving eight walnut halves, chop the remainder and stir into one of the bowls together with the tarragon.

Peel the pears carefully and cut in half. Remove the cores and hollow out four of the halves to make room to anchor the filling. Slice the other four halves and brush over with the lemon juice, pouring any remaining juice over them.

Fill the hollowed-out cavities with the cheese and nut mixture and put onto four small dessert plates. Fan out the slices of pear on each of the four plates as attractively as you can.

Gradually whisk the remaining yoghurt into the rest of the cheese in the second bowl, add the vinegar and mix to make a smooth dressing. Pour the dressing carefully over the sliced pears on the plates. Roughly chop the reserved walnuts and sprinkle over the top. Garnish the plates with the watercress and tarragon sprigs.

MAIN COURSE – TROUT WITH LIMES AND RED PEPPER

1 large red onion
1 red pepper
2 tbsp olive oil
1 dsp sherry vinegar
juice of 2 limes
3 tbsp fresh chopped parsley
2 dashes Tabasco sauce
4 small trout, gutted and cleaned
salt and freshly ground black pepper
watercress and quartered limes to garnish

For the sauce

1 large ripe avocado
1 tbsp natural yoghurt

Peel and slice the onion as thinly as possible. De-seed and dice the pepper into fairly small chunks. Heat the oil in a pan and fry the onion together with the sherry vinegar for 5 minutes. Add the pepper and cook for a further 2 minutes. Now add the juice of one of the limes, 2 tbsp of the parsley and the Tabasco. Mix thoroughly and remove from the heat.

Brush an oven-proof dish with a little oil and put in the fish. Season lightly and cover with the vegetable mixture. Tightly cover the dish with foil and bake in a moderate oven for about 20 minutes or until the fish is cooked through.

Halve the avocado and remove the stone and the skin, scraping well to remove all the bright green flesh clinging to the skin. Liquidise the flesh together with the juice of the remaining lime and the yoghurt.

Dish a trout onto each serving plate and sprinkle over the reserved parsley. Garnish with the watercress and two lime quarters. Spoon a quarter of the sauce on to each plate and serve with a large, fresh mixed green salad.

ENTERTAINING ON THE DIET

DESSERT – NORMANDY TRIFLE

900g cooking apples
1 lemon
115g sugar
175g trifle sponge cakes
2 tbsp apricot jam
3 tbsp Calvados (or other liqueur)
150ml apple juice
350g thick Greek yoghurt
1 red apple – Discovery would be a good choice
2 tbsp lemon juice
fresh mint

Peel and core the apples and cut roughly into chunks.
Grate the lemon rind and squeeze the juice. Over gentle
heat cook the apples, rind and lemon juice together until
soft. Add the sugar and mix well until smooth. Cool and
refrigerate.

Cut the sponge cakes in half and spread with the jam.
Now cut each cake into four. Lay out half the sponge
cakes in an attractive glass serving bowl. Mix together
the Calvados and apple juice and spoon half of it over
the sponge cakes. Now spread with half the remaining
apples and half the remaining sponge and juice.
Continue with the remaining apple, sponge and juice.
Cover and refrigerate for a few hours or overnight.

When ready to serve spread the yoghurt over the top.
Slice the red apple, brush well with the lemon juice and
pile in the middle. Decorate with mint leaves.

Did you know...?
In ancient times, the Chinese
referred to watercress as
'The Vegetable of the
Western Oceans'.

DINNER PARTY 3

(FOR 4 PEOPLE) – 890 CALORIES

STARTER – TOMATO AND BASIL SOUP

900g ripe tomatoes
2 large cloves garlic
2 tbsp olive oil
2 tbsp tomato purée
725ml vegetable stock
1 tsp sugar
40g small pasta shapes
1 bunch fresh basil
salt and freshly ground black pepper

Roughly chop the tomatoes. Slice the garlic cloves. Heat the oil in a pan and gently sauté the sliced garlic for about 2 minutes, being careful not to burn it. Add the roughly chopped tomatoes, the tomato purée, the stock and the sugar. Bring to the boil, reduce the heat and simmer for about 20 minutes.

Cook the pasta shapes in boiling, salted water until tender. Drain and keep to one side in cold water.

Liquidise the tomato mixture in a food processor and then pass through a sieve. Drain the pasta and add to the soup. Re-heat gently and stir in the finely chopped basil. Season to taste and serve at once.

MAIN COURSE – STUFFED PORK TENDERLOIN WITH ORANGE SAUCE

450g pork tenderloin
5 tsp vegetable oil
3 sheets filo pastry
watercress to garnish

For the filling

50g dried apricots
50g bacon
1 small onion
1 tbsp vegetable oil
1 tbsp fresh chopped parsley
15g pistachio nuts
50g fresh breadcrumbs

For the sauce

1 orange
450ml vegetable stock
2 tsp arrowroot
1 tbsp water
2 spring onions
1 tbsp Cointreau
1 tsp lemon juice
salt and freshly ground black pepper

Trim the tenderloin and make a deep cut along the length of the meat without going right through. Open out the meat and place on a length of clingfilm, putting another length of film over the top. Using a wooden meat mallet or rolling pin, bat out the meat until very thin, starting from the centre and batting to each end.

Soak the apricots, if necessary, in boiling water. Chop the bacon and the onion quite finely. Heat the oil in a pan and sauté the onion for about 4 minutes and then add the bacon and cook for a further 4 minutes, stirring continuously. Chop the parsley, pistachio nuts and apricots finely and add to the pan together with the breadcrumbs. Season with salt and pepper.

Uncover the tenderloin and lay the stuffing along its length. Fold the ends in and then the sides enclosing the stuffing. Tie securely, at intervals, with string.

Heat 3 tsp of the oil in a frying pan and seal over a high heat. Ensure that all sides of the meat are well sealed. Leave to cool for about 1 hour and then very carefully remove the string.

Very lightly oil the filo pastry and lay the sheets on top of each other and place the pork on the top. Fold over the ends and roll the meat in the pastry. Place on a lightly oiled non-stick baking tray and brush the pastry with the remaining oil and sprinkle with water. Bake in a pre-heated hot oven for about 30 minutes until the pastry is crisp and golden.

To make the sauce, pare the orange rind and cut finely into matchstick strips and set aside. Squeeze the juice from the orange and put into a small pan together with the stock. Bring to the boil and continue to cook, uncovered, until the sauce has reduced to about 285ml.

Mix the arrowroot with 1 tbsp of cold water and stir into the sauce. Stir until thickened. Now slice the spring onions finely and add to the sauce together with the liqueur, the lemon juice and the orange zest. Simmer for 2 minutes, season and put in a warm sauce boat.

Using a sharp knife, slice the meat and divide between four heated plates. Spoon some of the sauce on to each plate and garnish with the watercress. Serve with a green vegetable of your choice.

DESSERT – RASPBERRY FLUMMERY – SERVES 6

115g rolled oats
225g thick Greek yoghurt
2 tbsp clear honey
1 tbsp Drambuie or whisky
175g fresh raspberries

Spread the oats out evenly on an ungreased baking sheet and bake in a hot oven for about 4 minutes until they are pale golden brown. Allow to cool and place in a large bowl. Add the yoghurt, honey and whisky. Mix well together and put to chill for 1 hour.

Spoon the mixture into glass coupes, smooth over the tops and divide the raspberries on top. Decorate with mint sprigs.

Did you know...?
In the nineteenth century,
watercress was used as a
hangover cure!

DINNER PARTY 4

(FOR 4 PEOPLE) – 1015 CALORIES

STARTER – LOW-FAT WALDORF SALAD

350g celery
75g shelled walnut halves
3 crisp red apples
juice of 1 small lemon
50g sultanas
1 large lettuce heart

For the dressing

4 tbsp fromage frais
1 tbsp lemon juice
1 tbsp mayonnaise
1 tbsp walnut oil
salt and freshly ground black pepper

Mix the dressing ingredients together and season. Beat well until the mixture is thick and smooth.

String the celery stalks of course outer strings and slice. Reserve a few leaves for the garnish. Toast the walnuts lightly, cool and roughly chop 60g of them. Quarter and core the apples, leaving on the skin and slice. Put into a bowl and mix well with the lemon juice. Add the celery, walnuts and sultanas to the bowl. Taste and adjust the seasoning.

Line four bowls with the lettuce leaves, divide the salad between the bowls and pour over the dressing. Garnish with the remaining walnuts and the reserved celery leaves. Serve at once.

ENTERTAINING ON THE DIET

MAIN COURSE – GUINEA FOWL WITH RED CABBAGE

2 tbsp extra virgin olive oil
2 guinea fowl
2 medium onions, finely chopped
2 shallots, finely chopped
1 small red cabbage, finely shredded
75g raisins
6 juniper berries
2 large pieces orange peel
2 large sprigs thyme
150ml chicken stock
salt and freshly ground black pepper
1 tbsp white wine vinegar
watercress to garnish

Heat the olive oil in a flameproof casserole and brown the birds on all sides over a moderate to high heat. Remove and put to one side.

Add the onions and shallots to the casserole. Lower the heat and cook gently for about 5 minutes. Add the red cabbage to the onions together with the raisins. Mix well and cook for a further 5 minutes, stirring frequently.

Pre-heat the oven to 180°C. Crush the juniper berries and add to the pan with the orange peel and the thyme. Pour over the stock and season. Place both the fowl on top of the cabbage and cover. Cook in the oven for $1\frac{1}{2}$ hours.

Remove the birds and cut into four, discarding the back bone. Add the vinegar to the cabbage and adjust the seasoning. Dish the cabbage on to a warmed dish and arrange the joints on the top. Garnish with the watercress and serve with a large mixed green salad, dressed with a low-fat dressing.

DESSERT – FLORIDA COCKTAIL IN A SCENTED HONEY DRESSING

1 white grapefruit
1 ruby grapefruit
1 large orange
2 blood oranges
1 lime
mint sprigs to garnish

For the dressing

6 green cardamom pods
6 tbsp clear honey
2 tbsp rose-water

Pod and crush the cardamom seeds. Put all the ingredients for the dressing into a small pan and stir over a moderate heat for 2 minutes. Pour into a dish and leave to cool.

Peel all the fruit removing the peel and pith together. Release the segments by cutting each side of the membranes. It is important for the appearance of the dish that the fruit slices are neat. Arrange the slices around four plates, placing the grapefruit and orange slices alternately. Put the blood orange slices in the middle and put one segment of lime on the top. Pour over the dressing and chill. Garnish with sprigs of mint before serving.

Did you know...?
For every 100g of watercress
that you eat, you are
consuming approximately
66mg of Vitamin C.

DINNER PARTY 5

(FOR 4 PEOPLE) – 1047 CALORIES

ENTERTAINING ON THE DIET

STARTER – AVOCADO AND ORANGE SALAD

3 large oranges
½ cucumber
2 medium avocados
watercress

For the dressing

3 tbsp fresh orange juice
1 tbsp red wine vinegar
1 tsp grain mustard
1 tbsp extra virgin olive oil
2 tsp chives, finely snipped
salt and freshly ground black pepper

Slice away the peel and pith from the oranges. Do this over a bowl, reserving any juice. Peel the cucumber and cut in half lengthways removing the seeds with a teaspoon. Cut the avocado in half and remove the stone and the skin. Dice the flesh neatly.

Mix the dressing ingredients well together with the orange juice. Add the avocado and turn gently in the dressing, coating it well.

Arrange the orange slices and cucumber on individual plates as attractively as possible and spoon the avocado in the middle. Spoon over the rest of the dressing and garnish with the watercress.

MAIN COURSE – SKATE WING WITH TARRAGON SAUCE

900g skinned skate wing
175ml water
115ml dry white wine
½ lemon
1 small onion
3 tarragon stalks
6 peppercorns
½ tsp salt
watercress for garnish

For the sauce

1 lemon
1 tbsp tarragon, chopped
4 tbsp extra virgin olive oil
salt and freshly ground black pepper
2 dashes of Tabasco sauce
1 generous pinch caster sugar

Wash the skate and dry with kitchen paper. Cut into four equal portions. Pour 175ml of water and the wine into a pan large enough to hold the skate separately. Remove the peel from the ½ lemon in large strips, avoiding as much pith as possible and squeeze the juice into a bowl. Peel and chop the onion. Add the lemon rind and juice, onion, tarragon stalks, peppercorns and salt to the pan, and bring slowly to the boil.

Add the portions of skate, cover the pan and simmer gently for about 15 minutes or until the skate is cooked through.

In the meantime, to make the sauce, squeeze the juice out of the lemon and combine all the remaining ingredients in a small pan. Heat gently for 2 minutes and whisk thoroughly.

Lift the skate out of the pan with a fish slice. Arrange on four warmed dinner plates, spoon over the dressing and garnish with the watercress. Serve immediately, perhaps with green beans and tiny new potatoes sprinkled with chopped chives.

Did you know...?
Watercress is not just a brilliant aid to slimming. The Vitamins C and E, plus all the iron it contains, mean that it's fantastically good for your skin as well.

DESSERT – BAKED BANANAS

4 bananas
20g brown sugar
1 tbsp water
30ml brandy
60g butter
100g whipping cream

Pre-heat the oven to 180°C, and bake the bananas for 10 minutes until soft.

Melt the sugar in a pan with 1 tbsp water, add the butter and the brandy and heat through. Pour over the sugar mixture and serve with the whipped cream.

DINNER PARTY 6

(FOR 4 PEOPLE) – 910 CALORIES

STARTER – PRAWN AND PEACH COCKTAIL

2 large peaches
2 limes
1/2 sweet red pepper
1/2 sweet yellow pepper
1 tsp red chilli, finely chopped
2 tbsp fresh coriander, chopped
225g peeled prawns
2 tbsp extra virgin olive oil
1 little gem lettuce

Remove the stones from the peaches and chop finely. Squeeze the juice from the lime and core and dice the peppers. Put the peaches, lime juice, peppers, chopped chilli and coriander in a bowl, then add the prawns and chill for 2 hours.

Drain the liquid and mix it with the olive oil to make a dressing. Wash, dry and shred the lettuce and arrange in your serving bowls. Spoon over the prawn mixture and garnish with the remaining lime, scored and cut into four.

Did you know...?
Hippocrates, the 'father of modern medicine' is said to have chosen the site for his hospital because it was close to a stream where watercress grew in abundance.

MAIN COURSE – SPATCHCOCKED POUSSIN WITH CHILLI

4 poussins
lemon wedges and watercress for garnish

For the stuffing

2 red peppers
2 small onions
3 cloves garlic
2 teaspoons chilli powder (to taste)
3 tbsp extra virgin olive oil
salt

Cut down each side of the birds' backbones to remove them. Lay the poussins down on a board and press on the breastbone to flatten them.

Carefully loosen the skin from the flesh right across the breast, and a little way down the thighs, taking care not to tear it, ready for the stuffing.

Halve, de-seed and roughly chop the peppers. Peel and roughly chop the onions and crush the garlic. Liquidise all the stuffing ingredients except the oil in a food processor. When puréed, add the oil slowly while the processor is running until the mixture is quite smooth.

Spoon a quarter of the stuffing between the flesh and skin of each bird, smoothing evenly. Refrigerate for 4 hours, or preferably overnight.

Grill the poussins slowly until cooked through and golden brown. Garnish with the watercress add lemon wedges and serve with a large mixed green salad and a tomato and basil salad.

DESSERT – HOT RASPBERRY SOUFFLÉ

575g fresh raspberries, or thawed frozen raspberries
175g caster sugar
1 tbsp Kirsch
1 tsp icing sugar
5 egg whites (size 2)

Hull the raspberries – remove the stalks and the central core of the raspberry should come out with them – then liquidise them and push them through a sieve to remove the seeds. Reserve 285ml of the purée and stir 1 tbsp of the caster sugar into the remainder together with the Kirsch for the sauce.

Butter a 165 x 80mm soufflé dish and coat evenly with 1 tbsp of caster sugar. Whisk the egg whites until they hold their shape, then gradually whisk in the remaining caster sugar, whisking well between each addition until stiff and shiny.

In a large bowl fold a quarter of the egg whites into the reserved raspberry purée until well mixed, then gently fold in the rest of the egg whites, taking care not to beat any air out of them. Spoon the soufflé mixture into the prepared dish and mark a deep swirl in the top. Cook in the centre of the oven for 25–30 minutes, until well risen, but do not open the oven door during cooking.

Meanwhile, warm the sauce in a small pan, ready to serve in a small jug. Remove the soufflé from the oven and sift icing sugar over the top. Serve immediately with the hot raspberry sauce.

Did you know...?

Watercress contains not one but two powerful anti-cancer substances.

part **5**

dieting tips

So you've done it! If you've followed the instructions in this book, you've lost several pounds using the Watercress Soup Diet, continued your weight-loss, and trained your body to enjoy a healthier, more delicious way of eating. Congratulations!

You can, of course, return to the Watercress Soup Diet whenever you feel like it, provided you leave at least four weeks between each time you use it. In the meantime, here are fifty indispensable dieters' tips that will help consolidate the new you, and make your life as a slimmer just that little bit easier. The first section deals with dietary and lifestyle advice, the second provides suggestions for slimming down your appearance if you're still struggling to shed those extra pounds....

1.   Before eating or drinking anything else in the morning, drink a large glass of warm water. This is wonderful for your digestive system. Get into the habit of having a bottle of water at your point of work, in your car and on your bedside table, and drink copiously whenever you feel like eating outside the diet.

2.   Don't miss meals in order to lose weight. If you skip a meal, your blood sugar level drops and this leads to cravings for high-energy foods such as chocolate and sweets. Missing meals can also lead to bad long-term eating habits.

3.   Keep a covered dish of celery and/or cucumber sticks in the fridge to nibble when hunger bites.

4.   Always grill or steam food instead of frying. Always remove skin from chicken or buy skinless breasts so that you are not tempted. Choose very lean meat and white fish.

5.   Always choose the low-fat option when buying spreads, cheese or yoghurts.

6.   Before you start the diet, rid your fridge of butter, cream, bacon and full-fat cheese.

7.   Avoid second helpings. Eating less is the most important aid to weight loss.

8.   Try to keep yourself occupied. You forget to feel

hungry when you are absorbed in an interest or hobby or even your regular work.

9. Walk as much as you can. Avoid escalators and take the stairs. Make time to do some exercises every day.

10. Do everything you can to improve the way you feel about yourself. A new hairdo, new make-up or some more flattering clothes will do wonders for your self-esteem and speed you on your way to a newer, slimmer you.

11. Avoid eating too many calories in the evening, when there is less likelihood of burning them off. What the body cannot use will be stored as fat.

12. If you get hungry between meals, eat some fruit or raw vegetables. If you get too hungry you are more likely to eat too much later.

13. Good non-stick woks or frying pans use very little oil, so are a great advantage to the dieter.

14. Try making your own ice-cream using low-fat milk or yoghurt

15. Cook vegetables and fish in your microwave without the use of butter or oil.

16. Buy less red meat and then do so only when it is very lean, such as fillet of beef with all fat removed or pork tenderloin.

17. If you eat game, choose meat that is very low in fat, such as venison.

18. Don't eat too much cheese, and only use low-fat varieties. Remember, you can use less of a stronger-tasting cheese.

19. Drink less alcohol. Instead of two glasses of wine,

drink one. Spritzers are a great help, using half wine and half soda. Drink a spicy tomato juice or vegetable juice instead of an alcoholic aperitif. Drink lots of water and unsweetened fruit juices.

20. Use low-fat yogurt mixed with horseradish sauce or chives on your baked potato, or even cottage cheese with the same treatment.

21. Concentrate on fruit-based puddings and avoid chocolate and cream-based ones. A variety of fresh fruit, peeled, sliced and attractively displayed on a large platter would be delicious. For something special you could sprinkle over some liqueur, or otherwise lime or lemon juice.

22. Have realistic goals and allow for a few minor setbacks.

23. You may become discouraged if you reach a plateau after dieting for some time. This is when you need to drop your calorie allowance again or take more exercise. This should get the weight moving again.

24. Exercise boosts your energy for long days. If you think you are too tired, make yourself do just five minutes instead of half an hour. Once you start you will probably want to do more.

25. Researchers have found that walking for an hour a day decreases the risk of colon cancer by half. Walking speeds digested food through the body.

26. Use a skipping rope to make exercise more fun. Try to remember the skipping jingles you sang as a child – these should soon set you panting!

27. Avoid fizzy drinks. Even low-calorie drinks can give you a false, bloated appearance.

28. You can eat some vegetables to your heart's content – choose them from the Watercress Soup Diet Vegetable List. When you need to re-fuel between meals, fill up on green beans, broccoli, carrots, spinach, celery, mushrooms and lettuce.

29. Biscuits are really taboo when dieting. But if your body is screaming for a little treat, then one small wholemeal biscuit will satisfy your craving. Do not be tempted to eat any more – it will only make you feel worse.

30. When you go food shopping, always have a list and stick to it. Walk past all those temptations with gritty determination. You really can survive without them.

31. When you are eating a meal, put your knife and fork down every now and then and take a short rest. If you eat too quickly you cannot savour your food – learn to enjoy it.

32. Drink at least eight glasses of water per day.

33. Weigh yourself regularly and as soon as you put on some weight be sure to tackle it at once, before it increases.

34. Bars of frozen fruit juice are a good way of allowing yourself a little sweet treat.

35. Use mustard instead of mayonnaise in your sandwich.

36. Use wine vinegar or sushi vinegar in your salad instead of vinaigrette.

37. When a recipe calls for sugar, decreasing it by 25 per cent will not make any difference to its taste. Most of us are learning to prefer less sweet foods.

Follow the suggestions above and you'll soon be the owner of a slimline body. But cutting down on fatty food isn't the only way to give yourself a slimmer appearance. Here are a few pointers towards disguising those few extra pounds until they're gone for good.

38. Darker colours are more flattering to those attempting to slim, and wearing one colour from shoulder to shoe helps to streamline the body.

39. If you are top heavy, avoid breast pockets and double-breasted jackets, both of which broaden the body's appearance.

40. Avoid large flowery prints – these do not flatter you if you need to lose a few pounds.

41. A long jacket will hide a multitude of sins!

42. If you have a thick neck, wear V-necklines. They will create the illusion of a longer, slimmer body.

43. Delicate shoes make thick ankles look thicker – wear something a bit sturdier, with a good heel.

44. Hide heavy thighs with an A-line skirt.

45. A thick waist can be hidden by wearing a loosely fitting waistcoat.

46. Make sure that your clothes fit properly. Bulges are emphasised by wearing clothes that are too small.

47. Pay attention to your posture. Stand tall and enjoy

wearing your clothes!

48. A round face can be lengthened by creating a wispy fringe. The shortest part of the fringe should be at the centre of the forehead.

49. Upswept hair with loose tendrils will take attention away from the body.

50. Add height to the crown of your head and it will immediately lengthen your face.

index

	Day 1	Day 2	Day 3	Day 4	Day 5	Day 6	Day 7
Watercress Soup	Unlimited	Unlimited	Unlimited	Unlimited	Unlimited	Unlimited	Unlimited
Fruit from the WSD Fruit List	Unlimited		Unlimited				Unlimited
Vegetables from the WSD Vegetable List		Unlimited	Unlimited			Unlimited	Unlimited
Low-fat Yoghurt or Skimmed Milk (ml)	25 25 25 25 25 25 / 25 25 25 25 25 25	25 25 25 25 25 / 25 25 25 25 25	25 25 25 25 25 / 25 25 25 25 25	250 250 250 250 250 / 250 250 250 250 250	25 25 25 25 25 / 25 25 25 25 25	25 25 25 25 25 / 25 25 25 25 25	25 25 25 25 25 / 25 25 25 25 25
Bananas				1 2 3 4 5			
Baked Potato		1 Large Baked Potato					
Fish					Unlimited	Unlimited	
Chicken					Unlimited	Unlimited	
Tomatoes					1 2 3 4 5 6	Unlimited	

	Day 1	Day 2	Day 3	Day 4	Day 5	Day 6	Day 7
Watercress Soup	Unlimited	Unlimited	Unlimited	Unlimited	Unlimited	Unlimited	Unlimited
Fruit from the WSD Fruit List	Unlimited		Unlimited				Unlimited
Vegetables from the WSD Vegetable List		Unlimited	Unlimited			Unlimited	Unlimited
Low-fat Yoghurt or Skimmed Milk (ml)				250 250 250 250 250			
Bananas				1 2 3 4 5			
Baked Potato		1 Large Baked Potato					
Fish					Unlimited	Unlimited	
Chicken					Unlimited	Unlimited	
Tomatoes					1 2 3 4 5 6	Unlimited	

	Day 1	Day 2	Day 3	Day 4	Day 5	Day 6	Day 7
Watercress Soup	Unlimited	Unlimited	Unlimited	Unlimited	Unlimited	Unlimited	Unlimited
Fruit from the WSD Fruit List	Unlimited		Unlimited				Unlimited
Vegetables from the WSD Vegetable List		Unlimited	Unlimited			Unlimited	Unlimited
Low-fat Yoghurt or Skimmed Milk (ml)	25 25 25 25	25 25 25 25	25 25 25 25	250 250 250 250	25 25 25 25	25 25 25 25	25 25 25 25
Bananas				1 2 3 4 5			
Baked Potato		1 Large Baked Potato					
Fish					Unlimited	Unlimited	
Chicken					Unlimited	Unlimited	
Tomatoes					1 2 3 4 5 6	Unlimited	

	Day 1	Day 2	Day 3	Day 4	Day 5	Day 6	Day 7
Watercress Soup	Unlimited	Unlimited	Unlimited	Unlimited	Unlimited	Unlimited	Unlimited
Fruit from the WSD Fruit List	Unlimited		Unlimited				Unlimited
Vegetables from the WSD Vegetable List		Unlimited	Unlimited			Unlimited	
Low-fat Yoghurt or Skimmed Milk (ml)				250			
Bananas				1 2 3 4 5			
Baked Potato		1 Large Baked Potato					
Fish					Unlimited	Unlimited	
Chicken					Unlimited	Unlimited	
Tomatoes					1 2 3 4 5 6	Unlimited	